Mediterranean Diet Cookbook

Learn in a Comprehensive Way About Mediterranean Diet With 50+ Recipes to Enjoy Healthy Food

Contents

Introduction

A Mediterranean diet may be right for you if you're searching for an eating plan to keep your heart healthy. The Mediterranean diet combines the fundamentals of healthy eating with Mediterranean flavors & cooking methods. The discovery that the Mediterranean countries, like Italy and Greece, had fewer deaths from coronary heart diseases than the United States & northern Europe sparked interest in the Mediterranean diet in the 1960s. Following studies, it was discovered that the Mediterranean diet's linked to a lower risk of cardiovascular disease. Dietary Guidelines for Americans recommend the Mediterranean diet as one of the plans of healthy eating to enhance health & prevent chronic diseases. World Health Organization recognizes it as healthy as well as a sustainable diet pattern, and the United Nations Educational, Scientific, & Cultural Organization recognizes it as an intangible cultural asset. The Mediterranean diet's a way of consuming food that's based on traditional cuisines of Mediterranean countries. Mediterranean diet is typically rich in whole grains, vegetables, fruits, beans, nuts and seeds, & olive oil, though there is no single definition.

Everyday consumption of fruits, vegetables, healthy fats and whole grains are the main components of the Mediterranean diet.

- Consumption of poultry, eggs. fish, and beans, on a weekly basis
- Consumption of dairy products in moderation
- Consumption of red meat should be limited.

Sharing the meals with the family along with friends, admiring red wine glass, & being active physically are all important aspects of the Mediterranean diet. Fruits, vegetables, nuts, herbs, whole grain and beans form the basis of the Mediterranean diet. Plant-based edibles are used to create meals. The Mediterranean Diet includes moderate quantities of poultry, dairy, and eggs, as well as seafood. Red meat, on the other hand, is only consumed on rare occasions. The Mediterranean diet relies heavily on healthy fats. They're consumed in place of less healthy fats like saturated & trans fats, which are linked to heart disease. In the Mediterranean diet, olive oil's the main source of the added fat. Monounsaturated fats, such as those found in olive oil, have been shown to lower the total cholesterol as well as low-density lipoproteins (or the "bad") cholesterol level. Monounsaturated fat can also be found in nuts & seeds. In the Mediterranean diet, also fish is very important. Fatty fish like herring, lake trout sardines, salmon, albacore tuna, and mackerel are high in fatty acids (omega-3), a form of polyunsaturated fats that may help the body reduce inflammation. Fatty acids (Omega-3) also aid in the reduction of triglycerides, blood clotting, & the prevention of stroke as well as heart failure. In the Mediterranean diet, red wine is usually consumed in moderation. Although some studies have linked alcohol to a lower risk of heart disease, it is far from risk-free. Based on potential health benefits, Dietary Guideline for Americans advise against starting drinking or even drinking more frequently.

More fruits & vegetables will be consumed if you adopt a Mediterranean diet. The target for 7-10 servings of fruits and vegetables per day. In addition, cereal, whole-grain bread, and pasta will be required. You can also play around with different whole grains like bulgur and faro. You'll need to start eating more healthy fats. When cooking, you should use olive oil instead of butter. Instead of margarine or butter, try dipping your bread in olive oil. You should also increase your seafood consumption. Fish can be eaten twice a week. Tuna, trout, herring salmon, and mackerel, whether fresh or packed in water, are all good choices. The Grilled fish is delicious and easy to clean up. Fish that is Deep-fried should be avoided. At the same time, you must cut back on red meat consumption. The meat will have to be replaced with poultry, fish, or beans. If you are eating meat, choose lean cuts and keep your portions small. You can, however, consume dairy products. Low-fat plain or Greek yogurt, as well as small quantities of a variety of cheeses, are recommended. Keep in mind that spices and herbs enhance flavor while reducing the salt's need. The Mediterranean diet's a delectable and nutritious way of life. Most people who adopt this eating style swear they will never eat in some other way again.

CHAPTER 1: Basics of Mediterranean Diet

The Mediterranean diet is a broad term that refers to the traditional eating habits of Mediterranean countries. There is no one-size-fits-all Mediterranean diet. The Mediterranean is bordered by at least 16 countries. It is because of differences in economy, ethnic background, culture, religion, geography and agricultural production, eating styles differ between these countries and even between regions within each country.

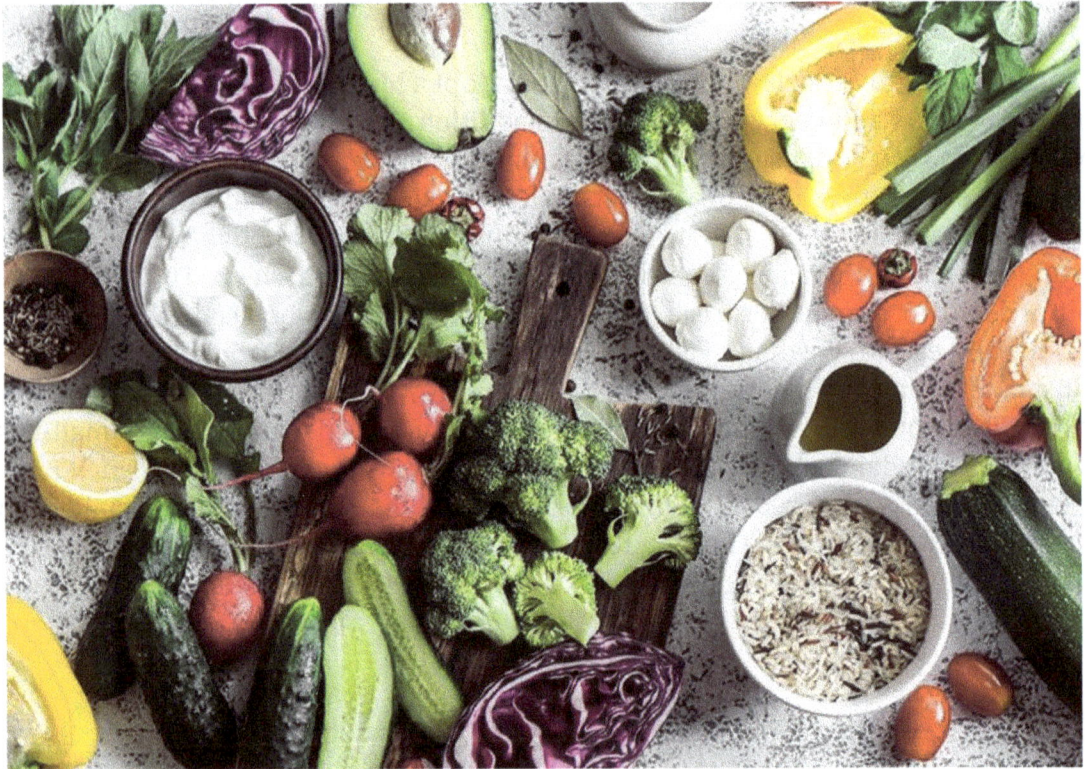

1.1 U.S. News Best Diet Rankings

Mediterranean Diet stood #1 in Best Diets Overall. A total of 39 diets were evaluated with feedback from a group of health experts. Mediterranean Diet is ranked:

#1 in Best Diets Overall

#1 in Best Heart-Healthy Diets (tie)

#1 in Best Diabetes Diets (tie)

#1 in Best Plant-Based Diets

#24 in Best Fast Weight-Loss Diets (tie)

You have to decide for yourself how many calories you must consume to maintain or lose your weight, how you'll stay active, & how you'll shape the Mediterranean menu because this is an eating pattern, not a structured diet. Mediterranean diet's pyramid can assist you in getting started. Fruits, vegetables, whole grains, olive oil, nuts, beans, legumes, flavorful herbs & spices; fish & seafood twice a week at least; poultry, cheese, eggs, & yogurt in moderation; and sweets & red meat like beef for the special occasions, according to the pyramid. Finish it with a splash of the red wine (only if desired) and some physical activity, and you're good to go. A glass of wine a day for the women & two glasses a day for the men is fine if the doctor says that. Red wine had gotten a raise because it has resveratrol, which is a compound that appears to extend life – but it would take 100s or even 1000s of glasses of wine to get sufficient resveratrol in order to make a difference.

1.2 Mediterranean Diet can help you lose weight

A Mediterranean diet may aid in weight loss. While few people believe that eating a Mediterranean-style diet, which is high in fats (imagine olive oil, avocado, olives, and cheese), will make them fat. However, more & more of the research is indicating that the opposite is correct. Naturally, it is dependent on what aspects that you adopt & how they compare to the current diet. Even If you include "calorie deficit" in your plan, such as eating lesser calories as compared to the daily recommended maximum or burning the extra calories through exercise, you should lose weight. It's entirely up to you how quickly & whether or not you keep those off.

1.3 How much should you exercise on Mediterranean Diet?

Exercise is required on the Mediterranean diet – but it doesn't have to feel like exercise.

Walking, often a central part of a Mediterranean lifestyle, is a good place to start, but add whatever you like into the mix – be it Jazzercise, gardening or Pilates.

Prime Reasons to Love the Mediterranean Diet

Given below are some of the prime reasons for loving and enjoying the Mediterranean diet.

No Calorie Counting

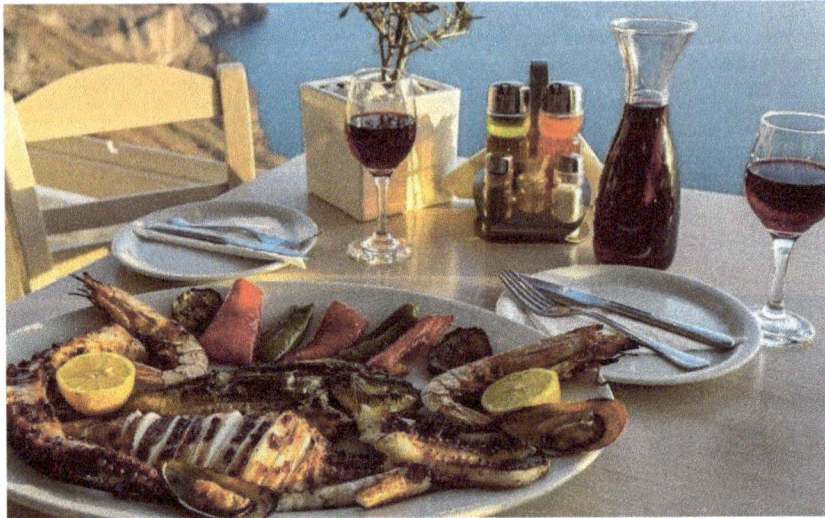

This meal plan does not require the use of a calculator. Rather than adding up numbers, you replace bad fats with heart-healthy fats. Instead of butter, use olive oil. Instead of red meat, try fish or poultry.

The food is also fresh

Mix cucumbers, spinach and tomatoes to make a delicious salad. Toss in some traditional Greek ingredients.

You can also eat bread

Go for a loaf that is made entirely of whole grains. It has more protein and minerals than white flour and is generally healthier.

Fat is also allowed in limited quantity

All you have to do now is look for the good kind. Olives, nuts and olive oil all contain it.

The menu is rich

There's a lot more to it than Greek and Italian food. Recipes from Turkey, Spain, Morocco and other countries are available. Choose foods that are simple to prepare.

It can be easily made

Mezzes are small, easy-to-assemble plates that are common in Greek cuisine. Arrange plates of olives, cheese and nuts, and you can also select a serve-it-cold casual meal for yourself.

You will not feel hungry

You'll have the opportunity to sample rich foods such as hummus, roasted sweet potatoes and the Lima Bean Spread.

Your heart will function properly

Nearly everything in the diet is heart-friendly. Nuts and olive oil can help lower "bad" cholesterol. Fruits, vegetables, and beans are all good for keeping arteries clear. Triglycerides, as well as blood pressure, are reduced by eating fish.

You will remain active

Your brain benefits from the same goodness that protects your heart. You do not eat foods like bad fats as well as processed foods. Antioxidant-rich foods, on the other hand, make this a brain-friendly eating style.

CHAPTER 2: Mediterranean Diet Breakfast Recipes

In this chapter, we have collected the most delicious Mediterranean diet recipes for your breakfast.

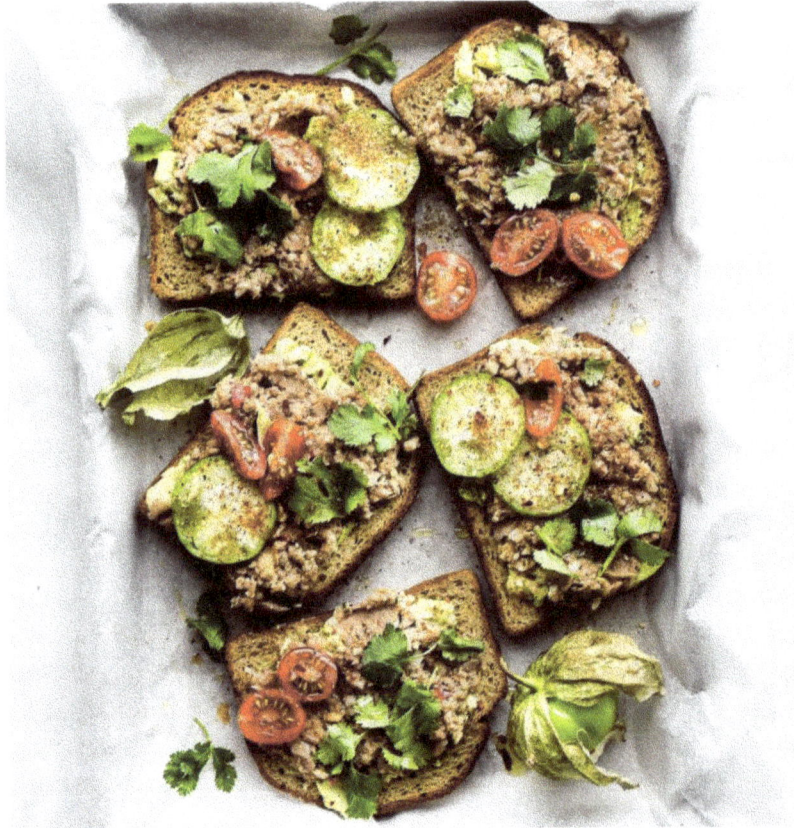

1. Balsamic Berries with Honey Yogurt

Preparation time

15 minutes

Servings

4 persons

Nutritional facts

111 calories

Ingredients

We have listed below the ingredients that are required for making this breakfast recipe:

- One cup blueberries
- 2 teaspoons honey
- One cup raspberries
- One tbsp balsamic vinegar
- 8 ounces strawberries, hulled and halved, or quartered if very large (about 1 1/2 cups)
- 2/3 cup whole-milk plain Greek yogurt
- 2 teaspoons honey

Instructions

You need to follow the under mentioned instructions for preparing this Mediterranean breakfast recipe:

1. In a large bowl, put the blueberries, the strawberries, and raspberries along with the balsamic vinegar. Let them sit for 10 minutes.
2. In a small bowl, stir the yogurt and honey together.
3. Divide the berries into glasses or serving bowls and apply a dollop of honey yogurt to each one.

2. Hearty Breakfast Fruit Salad

Preparation time

1 hour 15 minutes

Servings

4 persons

Nutritional facts

282 calories

Ingredients

We have listed below the ingredients that are required for making this breakfast recipe:

- half teaspoon kosher salt
- 1/2 large pineapple, peeled and cut into 1 1/2- to 2-inch chunks (2 to 2 1/2 cups)
- 6 medium tangerines or mandarins, or 5 large oranges (about 1 1/2 pounds total)
- 1 1/4 cups pomegranate seeds
- One cup pearl or hulled barley or any sturdy whole grain
- Three cups water
- Three tbsp olive or vegetable oil, divided

- half teaspoon kosher salt
- Quarter cup olive oil
- Quarter cup toasted hazelnut or nut oil
- 1 small bunch of fresh mint
- 1/3 cup honey or another sweetener
- Juice and finely grated zest of 1 lemon (about Quarter cup juice)
- Juice and finely grated zest of 2 limes (about Quarter cup juice)

Instructions

You need to follow the under mentioned instructions for preparing this Mediterranean breakfast recipe:

1. The two rimmed baking sheets are lined with parchment paper. Rinse The barley is then rinsed for approximately one minute in a strainer under cold water till the water below is clear. Then shake the strainer gently to drain off any excess water. Put the barley on one of the prepared baking sheets. Now take a spatula to spread out the grains into a single layer. Let it dry completely for around three to five minutes.

2. The water is then warmed in the microwave or on the stovetop. Then set aside.

3. Heat two tbsp of the oil in a medium pan at high heat till shimmering. The barley and toast are then added carefully, constantly stirring for about sixty to ninety seconds, till they just begin to darken a bit.

4. Insert the salt and the warm water. Then bring it to a boil. The heat is then reduced to the lowest or simmer your stovetop has. Then it is to be covered and cooked for forty to forty-five minutes till it turns soft and most of the liquid gets absorbed.

5. The pot is then removed from the heat. Allow it to stand, covered, for about ten minutes, allowing the barley steam and end water-absorption. In the process, prepare the mint, fruit and dressing.

6. Put the pineapple chunks into one of the large containers. The mandargins, tangerines or oranges are then peeled and sliced into small parts. You have to remove as much of the bitter white pith as you can. Put in another container. Cover that container and refrigerate. The pomegranate seeds are to be refrigerated separately in a covered container.

7. Then the mint leaves are thinly sliced or minced. Refrigerate these in a covered container.

8. Mix the salt, honey and juice and zest together in a medium bowl. Put the nut oil and the olive oil while mixing continuously till incorporated. Then it is covered and refrigerated in a jar.

9. The cooked barley is then transferred to the second prepared baking sheet. Then it is spread into a uniform layer. Allow it to cool completely for about ten to twenty minutes. Use the remaining one tbsp of oil for drizzling on the barley. Then mix it to coat.

10. Move the barley into a large container. Then cover it and refrigerate.

11. You can serve by scooping a two-thirds cup of the barley into every bowl. Then you can insert around ten to twelve orange pieces, about 6 pieces of pineapple and a quarter cup of pomegranate seeds into each bowl. Insert one to two tbsp of the mint into every bowl. Also, add two to three tbsp of the dressing to each bowl. If required, you can whisk the dressing. Stir to mix well and coat with the dressing.

3. Mediterranean Breakfast Sandwiches

Preparation time

20 minutes

Servings

4 persons

Nutritional facts

242 calories

Ingredients

We have listed below the ingredients that are required for making this breakfast recipe:

- Four multigrain sandwich thins
- Four teaspoons olive oil
- One tbsp snipped fresh rosemary, or half teaspoon dried rosemary, crushed
- Four eggs
- two cups fresh baby spinach leaves
- 1 medium tomato, cut into 8 thin slices
- Four tablespoons reduced-fat feta cheese
- one-eighth teaspoon kosher salt
- One pinch Freshly ground black pepper

Instructions

You need to follow the under mentioned instructions for preparing this Mediterranean breakfast recipe:

1. Heat oven to 375 degrees F. Slice sandwich into thin pieces. Then take two tsp of the olive oil for brushing of cut sides. Put on baking sheet. Toast for around five minutes in the oven or till edges turns light brown and crisp.

2. In the meantime, heat the 2 teaspoons of olive oil along with the rosemary in a large skillet over medium-high heat. Start breaking eggs, one at a time, and put the eggs into a skillet. It should be cooked for around one minute or till whites are set, but yolks are still runny. Use a spatula to break yolks. Flip eggs. The other side is to be cooked till done. It should then be removed from heat.

3. The bottom halves of the toasted sandwich thins are placed on four serving plates. Then spinach is to be distributed evenly on sandwich thins on plates. Each slice is to be topped with two of the tomato slices, one tbsp of the feta cheese and an egg. Then use salt and pepper as per taste. Finally, it is to be topped with the remaining sandwich thin halves.

4. The Best Shakshuka

Preparation time

40 minutes

Servings

4 persons

Nutritional facts

146 calories

Ingredients

We have listed below the ingredients that are required for making this breakfast recipe:

- Two tbsp tomato paste
- One tbsp harissa
- 3 cloves garlic, minced
- 2 ounces feta cheese, crumbled (about 1/2 cup, optional)
- 1 (28-ounce) can whole peeled tomatoes
- Two tbsp olive oil
- 1 small yellow onion, finely chopped
- Crusty bread or pita, for serving (optional)
- One tsp ground cumin
- half teaspoon kosher salt
- 6 large eggs
- Quarter cup loosely packed chopped fresh cilantro leaves and tender stems

Instructions

You need to follow the under mentioned instructions for preparing this Mediterranean breakfast recipe:

1. Pour into a large bowl the tomatoes with their juices. Crush gently into bite-sized pieces with your hands; put aside.

2. Heat the oil over medium heat in a 10- or 12-inch skillet until it begins to shimmer. Insert the onion and sauté for 5 to 6 minutes till translucent and softened. Insert the harissa, the tomato paste, garlic, cumin and salt, and sauté for around 1 minute, until fragrant.

3. Insert the tomatoes, and get them to a simmer. Simmer gently for about 10 minutes until the sauce has thickened slightly.

4. Withdraw the skillet from the heat. In the sauce, make 6 little wells. Into each well, break an egg.

5. Spoon a little sauce gently over the egg whites, rendering the yolks exposed. This can help in getting the whites to cook swiftly.

6. Cover the skillet and return it to medium-low heat.

7. Cook, turning the pan as needed so that the eggs cook uniformly for 8 to 12 minutes until the whites are set, and the yolks are to the correct doneness (check on it a few times). When you shake the pan softly, the eggs should always jiggle in the center.

8. Remove from the heat. If used, sprinkle with cilantro and feta and, if desired, serve with bread or pita.

5. Spinach and Artichoke Frittata

Preparation time

30 minutes

Servings

4 persons

Nutritional facts

316 calories

Ingredients

We have listed below the ingredients that are required for making this breakfast recipe:

- Half cup sour cream (full-fat)
- olive oil, Two tbsp
- About fourteen ounces of marinated hearts of artichoke, drained, dried, & quartered
- Five ounces of baby spinach (almost 5 fully packed cups)
- Two minced cloves garlic,
- One tbsp dijon mustard

- Ten large eggs
- One tsp kosher salt
- Quarter tsp freshly ground black pepper
- One cup grated Parmesan cheese (about 3 ounces), divided

Instructions

You need to follow the under mentioned instructions for preparing this Mediterranean breakfast recipe:

1. In the center of the oven, arrange a rack and heat it to 400 ° F.
2. Put in a wide bowl the sour cream, eggs, mustard, pepper, salt and a half cup of the Parmesan and whisk to mix; set aside.
3. Heat the oil over medium heat in an oven-safe nonstick skillet or an oven. In a single layer, add the artichokes and fry, stirring regularly, till lightly browned, for 6 to 8 minutes. Insert the spinach and garlic and toss for about 2 minutes before the spinach is wilted and nearly all of the liquid has evaporated.
4. Spread it all into an even layer. Pour over the vegetables the egg mixture. Sprinkle with the remaining Parmesan Half Cup. To make sure that the eggs settle uniformly over all the vegetables, tilt the pan. Cook undisturbed, 2 to 3 minutes, till the eggs at the edges of the pan start to set.
5. Bake for 12 to 15 minutes until the eggs are totally set. Cut a little slit in the middle of the frittata to check. Bake for a few more minutes if the raw eggs run into the cut.
6. Let it cool for 5 minutes in the pan.
7. Serve warm and enjoy.

6. Mediterranean Breakfast Board

Preparation time

30 minutes

Servings

6-12 persons

Nutritional facts

220 calories

Ingredients

We have listed below the ingredients that are required for making this breakfast recipe:

- Feta cheese or 1 Labneh Recipe
- 1 Tabouli Recipe
- one Falafel Recipe

- one Classical Hummus Recipe (or the roast garlic hummus or red bell pepper hummus)
- one Baba Ganoush Recipe
- 1-2 sliced tomatoes,
- 1 sliced English cucumber,
- 6-7 Radish, sliced or halved
- Grapes (palette cleanser)
- Fresh herbs for garnish
- Assorted olive (I like a mix of green olives and kalamata olives)
- Marinated mushrooms or artichokes
- Evoo early harvest & za'atar
- Pita Bread, cut into quarters

Instructions

You need to follow the under mentioned instructions for preparing this Mediterranean breakfast recipe:

1. Make the falafel as per the instructions of the recipe. To soak the chickpeas, you'll need to move at least the night before. Make the hummus and baba ganoush as per the directions in this recipe. Both of these can be made the night before and stored in the refrigerator. To spice things up, try roasted garlic hummus as well as roasted red pepper hummus. (If you don't have time to make your own, use good store-bought hummus.)
2. Using this recipe, slice feta cheese or make Labneh ahead of time.
3. To make tabouli, follow this recipe. It's possible to make it ahead of time and keep it refrigerated in glass containers with tight lids.
4. Put the olive oil, hummus, baba ganoush, za'atar and tabouli in bowls to make the Mediterranean breakfast board. To create a focal point, but the largest bowl in the middle of a large wooden board and/or platter. To create movement and shape, assemble the remaining bowls on various parts of the board as well as the platter. Place the remaining ingredients, such as sliced vegetables, falafel, and pita bread, in the gaps between the bowls. If desired, garnish with fresh herbs and add grapes.

7. Caprese Avocado Toast

Preparation time

10 minutes

Servings

2 persons

Nutritional facts

649 calories

Ingredients

We have listed below the ingredients that are required for making this breakfast recipe:

- One Medium Halved Avocado & Pit Removed
- Two Tbsp Balsamic Glaze
- 8 Halved Grape Tomatoes,
- Two Ounces Ciliegine Fresh Or Mozzarella Balls, Bite-Sized (At Least 12)
- 2 Slices Of Sandwich Bread (Hearty), Like Peasant Bread, Whole-Wheat Sourdough, Or The Multi-Grain
- Four Big Basil Leaves, Freshly Torn

Instructions

You need to follow the under mentioned instructions for preparing this Mediterranean breakfast recipe:

1. Toast the bread. Mash in a small bowl the avocado while toasting the bread.
2. Over the bread, spread the mashed avocado. Top with the basil leaves, tomatoes and mozzarella balls each slice. Then sprinkle the balsamic glaze. Immediately serve.

8. Mediterranean Diet Mini Omelets

Preparation time

40 minutes

Servings

2-4 persons

Nutritional facts

185 calories

Ingredients

We have listed below the ingredients that are required for making this breakfast recipe:

- Olive oil – 2 teaspoons or as needed
- Chopped Vegetables- 1 cup
- Seasonings Salt and Pepper as per taste
- Eggs- 8
- Half and Half- ½ cup

- Cheese- ¼ cup

Instructions

You need to follow the under mentioned instructions for preparing this Mediterranean breakfast recipe:

1. Preheat the oven to 350 degrees Fahrenheit. Because this recipe is susceptible to sticking, grease your muffin pan or ramekins. You could also spray a little nonstick spray on top of it.

2. To make the dairy and eggs fluffy, whisk them together in a mixing bowl with a whisk. After that, add the cheese and any seasonings you want. Fold in any remaining vegetables or ingredients, then transfer the mixture evenly to the prepared ramekins or muffin pan.

3. Bake the omelets until they are firm to the touch. This could take anywhere from 25 to 30 minutes, depending on what you're baking them with. Remove from the oven and set aside for 5–10 minutes before serving.

9. Spinach Feta Breakfast Wraps

Preparation time

25 minutes

Servings

4 persons

Nutritional facts

543 calories

Ingredients

We have listed below the ingredients that are required for making this breakfast recipe:

- 1/2 pound (about 5 cups) baby spinach
- 4 whole-wheat tortillas (about 9 inches in diameter, burrito-sized)
- Butter or olive oil Salt
- Pepper
- 1/2 pint cherry or grape tomatoes, halved
- Ten large eggs
- 4 ounces feta cheese, crumbled

Instructions

You need to follow the under mentioned instructions for preparing this Mediterranean breakfast recipe:

1. Whisk the eggs in a large bowl until the whites and yolks are fully mixed. Over medium heat, put a large skillet and add ample butter or olive oil to cover the rim. Pour in the eggs when the butter is melted or when the oil is heated and stir regularly until the eggs are fried. Stir in a pinch of salt and a generous quantity of black pepper, then stir to cool to room temperature on a large plate.

2. Rinse the skillet or clean it down, bring it back over medium heat and apply yet another pat of butter or oil. Insert the spinach and cook until the spinach is only wilted, stirring occasionally. To cool to room temperature, spread the cooked spinach on another large plate.

3. Arrange a tortilla on aboard. In the center of the tortilla, add about a quarter of each of the eggs, spinach, tomatoes, and feta and cover them tightly. Repeat for the three tortillas that remain. In a gallon zip-top bag, put the wraps and freeze until ready to eat. Wrap the burritos in aluminum foil to avoid freezer burn when freezing for longer than a week.

10. Banana Split Yogurt

Preparation time

20 minutes

Servings

1 person

Nutritional facts

220 calories

Ingredients

We have listed below the ingredients that are required for making this breakfast recipe:

- 1-2 tsp strawberry jam
- 1-2tsp cacao nibs
- 1 cup plain Greek yogurt
- 1/2 banana, sliced

Instructions

You need to follow the under mentioned instructions for preparing this Mediterranean breakfast recipe:

1. Combine all ingredients in a bowl and serve.
2. Strawberry jam can be replaced with blueberry, raspberry or other flavors of jam.

11. Mediterranean Quinoa Salad

Preparation time

15 minutes

Servings

4 persons

Nutritional facts

483 calories

Ingredients

We have listed below the ingredients that are required for making this breakfast recipe:

- 1 tablespoon balsamic vinegar
- 1 15 ounces can garbanzo beans drained
- 1 package DeLallo Zesty Salad Savors
- 2 pressed garlic cloves
- half teaspoon dried minced basil
- half tsp dried thyme should be crushed between the fingers
- 1 1/2 cups dry quinoa
- kosher salt & black pepper freshly ground
- 1/2 teaspoon kosher salt
- 1/2 cup extra virgin olive oil
- 3 cups arugula

Instructions

You need to follow the under mentioned instructions for preparing this Mediterranean breakfast recipe:

1. Cook quinoa as directed on the package, adding 1/2 teaspoon salt to the water. Allow to cool completely.
2. Combine the balsamic vinegar, olive oil, pressed garlic, thyme and basil in a mixing bowl. Whisk everything together until it's smooth. Set aside after seasoning with the kosher salt as well as black pepper freshly ground.
3. Add the quinoa, arugula, garbanzo beans, and Salad Savors package contents to a big serving bowl (kalamata olives, red bell pepper & feta cheese).
4. Then drizzle the dressing over the salad and top with the basil. Season with salt and pepper to taste. Allow to cool before serving.

12. Mediterranean Breakfast Quesadillas
Preparation time

10 minutes

Servings

1 person

Nutritional facts

402 calories

Ingredients

We have listed below the ingredients that are required for making this breakfast recipe:

- 1/2 slices tomato,
- handful basil,
- pepper and salt to taste
- 2 eggs, cooked, scrambled
- 1/4 cup mozzarella
- one tortilla

Instructions

You need to follow the under mentioned instructions for preparing this Mediterranean breakfast recipe:

1. Scramble eggs, so don't let them overcook. Season to taste with salt & pepper.
2. On half of the tortilla, spread eggs. Sliced tomato, basil, & mozzarella cheese go on top.
3. Fold tortilla in half and toast all sides in an oiled skillet until lightly browned
4. Slice & serve right away, or snack when on the run.

13. Mediterranean Breakfast Tostadas

Preparation time

15 minutes

Servings

4 persons

Nutritional facts

828 calories

Ingredients

We have listed below the ingredients that are required for making this breakfast recipe:

- 1/2 c. red pepper, diced
- 1/2 c. tomatoes, diced
- 1/4 c. feta crumbled

- 1/2 c. green onions, chopped
- 8 eggs beaten
- 1/2 c. skim milk
- 4 tostadas
- 1/2 c. roasted red pepper hummus
- 1/2 tsp. garlic powder
- 1/2 tsp. oregano
- 1/2 c. cucumber, seeded and chopped

Instructions

You need to follow the under mentioned instructions for preparing this Mediterranean breakfast recipe:

1. Cook the red peppers in a large nonstick skillet at medium heat for 2-3 minutes or until softened. In a skillet, whisk together the eggs, milk, garlic powder, oregano, and green onions until the egg whites are no more translucent (approximately 2 minutes).
2. Tostadas should be topped with hummus, egg mixture, cucumber, tomatoes, and feta cheese. Serve right away.

14. Date & Pine Nut Overnight Oatmeal

Preparation time

Active 10 minutes

Servings

2 persons

Nutritional facts

282 calories

Ingredients

We have listed below the ingredients that are required for making this breakfast recipe:

- Pinch of salt
- 1 teaspoon honey
- 2 tablespoons chopped dates
- 1 tablespoon toasted pine nuts
- ½ cup old-fashioned rolled oats
- ½ cup water
- ¼ teaspoon ground cinnamon

Instructions

You need to follow the under mentioned instructions for preparing this Mediterranean breakfast recipe:

1. Stir together the oats, water as well as salt in a jar or bowl. Refrigerate overnight, covered.

2. If desired, heat the oats in the morning or eat them cold. Dates, pine nuts, honey, and cinnamon are sprinkled on top.

15. Spinach & Egg Scramble with Raspberries

Preparation time

10 minutes

Servings

1 person

Nutritional facts

296 calories

Ingredients

We have listed below the ingredients that are required for making this breakfast recipe:

- Pinch of ground pepper
- 1 slice whole-grain bread, toasted
- 1 tsp canola oil
- one ½ cups of baby spinach
- 2 big, lightly beaten eggs,
- Pinch of the kosher salt
- ½ cup fresh raspberries

Instructions

You need to follow the under mentioned instructions for preparing this Mediterranean breakfast recipe:

1. In a small nonstick skillet, heat the oil over medium-high heat. Cook, frequently stirring, until the spinach has wilted, about one to two minutes.

2. Place the spinach on a serving plate. Clean the pan, place it over medium heat, and crack the eggs into it. Cook, stirring either once or twice to ensure even cooking, for 1 to 2 minutes, or until just set. Add the spinach, salt, and pepper to taste. With toast and raspberries, serve the scramble.

16. Easy Homemade Muesli

Preparation time

15 minutes

Servings

5 persons

Nutritional facts

275 calories

Ingredients

We have listed below the ingredients that are required for making this breakfast recipe:

- Three and a half cup rolled oats
- Half cup wheat bran
- half teaspoon kosher salt
- half teaspoon ground cinnamon
- Half cup sliced almonds
- Quarter cup raw pecans, coarsely chopped
- Quarter cup dried apricots, coarsely chopped
- Quarter cup dried cherries
- Quarter cup raw pepitas (shelled pumpkin seeds)
- Half cup unsweetened coconut flakes

Instructions

You need to follow the under mentioned instructions for preparing this Mediterranean breakfast recipe:

1. Toast the grains, nuts, and seeds. Arrange 2 racks to divide the oven into thirds and heat to 350°F. Place the oats, wheat bran, salt, and cinnamon on a rimmed baking sheet; toss to combine; and spread into an even layer. Place the almonds, pecans, and pepitas on a second rimmed baking sheet; toss to combine; and spread into an even layer. Transfer both baking sheets to the oven, placing oats on the top rack and nuts on the bottom. Bake until nuts are fragrant, 10 to 12 minutes.

2. Add the coconut. Remove the baking sheet with the nuts and set it aside to cool. Sprinkle the coconut over the oats, return to the upper rack, and bake until the coconut is golden-brown, about 5 minutes more. Remove from oven and set aside to cool for about 10 minutes.

3. Transfer to a large bowl. Transfer the contents of both baking sheets to a large bowl.

4. Add the dried fruit. Add the apricots and cherries and toss to combine.

5. Transfer to an airtight container. Muesli can be stored in an airtight container at room temperature for up to 1 month.

6. Enjoy as desired. It can be enjoyed as cereal, oatmeal, with yogurt or overnight oats after topping with fresh fruit and a drizzle of maple syrup or honey if desired.

17. Kale and Goat Cheese Frittata Cups

Preparation time

55 minutes

Servings

4 persons

Nutritional facts

179 calories

Ingredients

We have listed below the ingredients that are required for making this breakfast recipe:

- Three tbsp olive oil
- Quarter tsp red pepper flakes
- half teaspoon dried thyme
- Quarter cup goat cheese, crumbled
- 8 large eggs
- Quarter tsp salt
- two cups chopped lacinato kale
- 1 garlic clove, thinly sliced
- Dash ground black pepper

Instructions

You need to follow the under mentioned instructions for preparing this Mediterranean breakfast recipe:

1. Heat the oven to 350°F. Remove the leaves from the ribs of the kale to get two cups of kale. Wash and dry the leaves and slice them into strips that are 1/2-inch wide.

2. Cook the garlic in a tablespoon of oil over medium-high heat for 30 seconds in a 10-inch nonstick skillet. Insert the kale and red pepper flakes and simmer for 1 to 2 minutes until wilted.

3. Beat the eggs in a medium bowl of salt and pepper. To the egg mixture, add the kale and thyme.

4. Use the remaining 2 tbsp of oil to grease 4 of the cups with a 4-cup muffin pan (you can also use butter or non-stick spray if you prefer). Sprinkle on the top of the goat cheese. Bake for about 25 to 30 minutes until they are set in the center.

5. Frittata is best eaten fresh from the oven or on the next day, but it is possible to keep leftovers in a refrigerator.

18. Easy and Fluffy Lemon Ricotta Cakes

Preparation time

28 minutes

Servings

4 persons

Nutritional facts

344 calories

Ingredients

We have listed below the ingredients that are required for making this breakfast recipe:

- One cup ricotta cheese whole-milk
- Quarter tsp kosher salt
- Unsalted butter for cooking
- Half cup whole or 2 % milk
- 4 large eggs
- 1 medium lemon
- One cup all-purpose flour
- One tbsp granulated sugar
- One tsp baking powder

For the topping: fresh berries, citrus segments, maple syrup or lemon curd,

Instructions

You need to follow the under mentioned instructions for preparing this Mediterranean breakfast recipe:

1. Separate 4 big eggs and put whites in a large bowl of the stand mixer equipped with whisk attachment & the yolks. (Alternatively, when you use an electric mixer or whisk by the hand with a powerful whisk, you may place the whites in a medium bowl.)

2. Finely grate one medium lemon zest onto egg yolks, and then squeeze the lemon juice into a bowl. It should be around one tbsp zest and three tbsp juice. Attach 1 cup of ricotta cheese (whole milk) and a half cup of whole milk or 2 % milk & whisk

to blend. Add one cup of flour, 1 tbsp of granulated sugar, one tsp of baking powder, & 1 tsp of kosher salt & whisk until mixed; try to avoid over mixing.

3. Beat egg whites at medium-high velocity for 2-3 minutes till stiff peaks develop. (Alternatively, beat using an electric mixer or strong whisk.) To lighten it, stir one-third of the pounded egg whites with a rubber spatula into the batter of egg yolk. Then, when just mixed, gently fold the rest of the egg whites in; do not over-mix.

4. Over medium fire, heat a broad griddle or nonstick skillet or cast iron. Apply to the skillet one teaspoon of unsalted butter and twist to coat. In Quarter Cup portions, drop batter into pan, 3 at once. Use the bottom of the measuring cup or spatula, if necessary, to spread each section gently into rough four-inch rounds. Then Cook for 2 to 3 minutes before bubbles emerge on the top, the edges start to look crispy, and bottoms are lightly browned. Flip pancakes & cook for 2 to 3 more minutes before the other side's golden-brown.

5. Move pancakes to an oven or the plate that is warm. Repeat cooking the remaining batter while using one tsp of butter for every batch and, if necessary, cleaning the skillet in batches. Serve pancakes promptly, with a preferable topping.

19. Smashed Eggs Toast with Herby Lemon Yogurt

Preparation time

20 minutes

Servings

4 persons

Nutritional facts

437 calories

Ingredients

We have listed below the ingredients that are required for making this breakfast recipe:

- 1 medium lemon
- Two tbsp finely chopped fresh basil leaves, plus more for garnish
- Two tbsp finely chopped fresh dill, plus more for garnish
- half teaspoon freshly ground black pepper, plus more for sprinkling
- 4 large slices of country or sourdough bread (about 1-inch thick)
- 4 tablespoons unsalted butter, divided
- Two tbsp finely chopped fresh chives, plus more for garnish
- 8 large eggs
- 1 clove garlic

- two cups plain Greek yogurt
- Two tbsp extra-virgin olive oil, plus more for drizzling
- 3/4 teaspoon kosher salt, plus more for sprinkling

Instructions

You need to follow the under mentioned instructions for preparing this Mediterranean breakfast recipe:

1. Fill a big pot with around 5 inches of water and bring it at high heat to a rolling boil; fill a large bowl of cold water and ice. Lower the heat until the water simmers easily. One at a time, softly lower eight large eggs into the water. For precisely six minutes and 30 seconds, boil. Move the eggs to the ice bath using a slotted spoon. Let the eggs remain for 2 minutes in the ice bath, then peel them underwater and set them aside.

2. Make the following by inserting these into a medium bowl: Mince 1 clove of garlic. Finely rub the zest 1 medium lemon, then add the lemon juice. Chop until you have two tablespoons of fresh basil leaves, two tablespoons of fresh dill, and two tablespoons of fresh chives. Apply two cups of Greek yogurt, two teaspoons of extra virgin olive oil, three-quarters of a teaspoon of kosher salt and half a teaspoon of black pepper. Stir to blend.

3. Cut 4 slices of crusty bread (1 inch thick). Melt 2 tablespoons of unsalted butter over medium heat in a large skillet. Insert 2 of the slices and fry, about 2 minutes on each side, until golden brown and crisp. Move it to a large dish. With the remaining two teaspoons of unsalted butter and bread, repeat.

4. Spread on the bread the yogurt mixture, then cover each toast with 2 of the eggs. Smash the eggs carefully with the back of a spoon. Sprinkle with black pepper, spices, and more kosher salt. You can drizzle with more olive oil.

20. Mediterranean Breakfast Pittas

Preparation time

25 minutes

Servings

4 persons

Nutritional facts

206 calories

Ingredients

We have listed below the ingredients that are required for making this breakfast recipe:

- 2 whole-wheat pita bread with pockets, cut in half
- Half cup hummus (4 ounces)

- Hot sauce (optional)
- 1 medium cucumber, thinly sliced into rounds
- 2 medium tomatoes, large dice
- A handful of fresh parsley leaves, coarsely chopped
- 4 large eggs, at room temperature
- Salt
- Freshly ground black pepper

Instructions

You need to follow the under mentioned instructions for preparing this Mediterranean breakfast recipe:

1. Fill with water a medium saucepan and bring it to a boil. Place the room-temperature eggs gently in the water. Then cook for 7 minutes. Drain the water. Then put the eggs under cold water. Peel the eggs and cut them into strips that are 1/4-inch thick. Sprinkle along with salt and then set aside with.

2. Spread the 2 tbsp of hummus within each pita bag. Add a few slices of cucumber and a few sliced tomatoes to each pita. Use salt and pepper to sprinkle. If you are using, sprinkle with parsley and hot sauce after tucking one sliced egg into each pita.

21. Crispy White Beans with Greens and Poached Egg

Preparation time

35 minutes

Servings

4 persons

Nutritional facts

301 calories

Ingredients

We have listed below the ingredients that are required for making this breakfast recipe:

- 1 (15-ounce) can cannellini beans, drained and rinsed
- One tsp kosher salt, divided
- One tbsp freshly squeezed lemon juice
- 4 large eggs, poached
- 2 teaspoons za'atar, divided

- 1 medium bunch Swiss chard (about 10 ounces), stems removed and leaves thinly sliced
- Three tbsp olive oil, divided
- 2 cloves garlic, minced
- Quarter tsp red pepper flakes, plus more for serving

Instructions

You need to follow the under mentioned instructions for preparing this Mediterranean breakfast recipe:

1. Heat two tablespoons of oil over medium-high heat until it shimmers in a large frying pan. Insert the beans, scatter into an even layer, and cook until the beans on the bottom are gently browned, 2 to 4 minutes, uninterrupted. Insert half a teaspoon of salt and a teaspoon of za'atar, and mix to combine. Spread the beans again and cook for 3 to 5 more minutes, stirring as required, till golden-brown and blistered on sides.

2. Apply the remaining tablespoon to the pan. Add the chard, the remaining half a teaspoon of salt, the remaining tsp za'atar, garlic, and flakes of red pepper. Cook, stirring regularly, for 3 to 5 minutes until the chard is wilted. To mix, remove the pan from the heat. Then add the lemon juice, and toss.

3. Divide the beans and greens into four bowls and finish each with a poached egg along with more flakes of red pepper. Serve it warm.

22. Breakfast Grain Salad with Blueberries, Hazlenuts and Lemon
Preparation time

40 minutes

Servings

5 persons

Nutritional facts

353 calories

Ingredients

We have listed below the ingredients that are required for making this breakfast recipe:

- Half cup dry millet
- Three tbsp olive oil, divided
- 1 (1-inch) piece fresh ginger, peeled and cut into coins
- 2 large lemons, zest and juice
- Half cup maple syrup

- One cup steel-cut oats
- two cups hazelnuts, roughly chopped and toasted
- two cups blueberries or mixed berries
- One cup dry golden quinoa
- One cup greek yogurt (or soy yogurt, if you want to make this vegan)
- Quarter tsp nutmeg

Instructions

You need to follow the under mentioned instructions for preparing this Mediterranean breakfast recipe:

1. In a fine-mesh strainer, combine the oats, quinoa, and millet and rinse them under running water for about a minute. And put aside.

2. Heat one tablespoon of oil over medium-high heat in a 3-quart saucepan. Add the rinsed grains and simmer for 2 to 3 minutes or until toasted. Throw in four and a half cups of water and add 3/4 of a teaspoon of cinnamon, ginger coins, and 1 lemon zest.

3. Boil, cover, turn the heat down and simmer for 20 minutes. Switch off the heat and let it sit for 5 minutes, then use a fork to loosen the lid and fluff. Get the ginger removed. On a large baking sheet, scatter the hot grains and allow them to cool for a minimum of thirty minutes.

4. Spoon the grains that are cooled into a large bowl. Stir in the second lemon's zest.

5. In a medium bowl, stir the remaining 2 tbsp olive oil until emulsified with the juice of both lemons. Add the yogurt, maple syrup and nutmeg to the whisk. Pour it onto the grains and swirl until the grains are well-coated. Stir in the hazelnuts and blueberries with the toasted ones. If required, test and season with additional salt.

6. Refrigerate overnight; the flavors actually come together in the refrigerator overnight.

CHAPTER 3: Mediterranean Diet Lunch Recipes

This chapter is a collection of the most delicious Mediterranean diet recipes for your lunch. These recipes shall protect you from high blood pressure, high cholesterol as well as obesity.

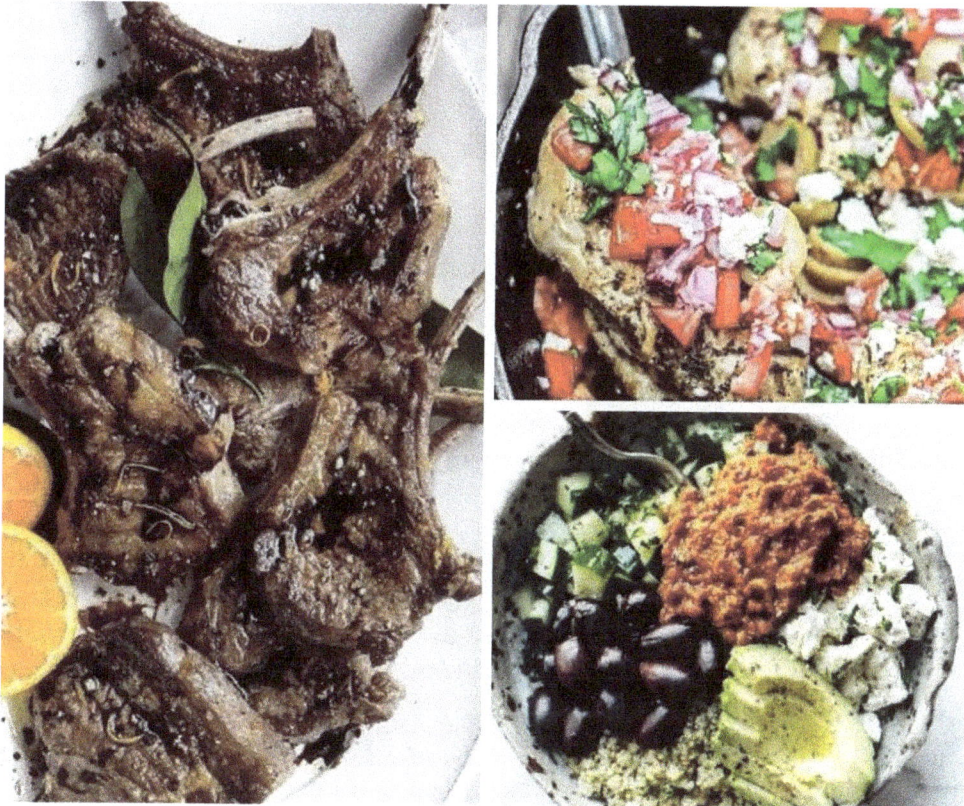

1. Greek Meatball Mezze Bowls

Preparation time

35 minutes

Servings

4 persons

Nutritional facts

392 calories

Ingredients

We have listed below the ingredients that are required for making this breakfast recipe:

- ½ tsp garlic powder

- half tsp oregano dried
- ⅜ divided teaspoon salt,
- ⅜ tsp divided ground pepper,
- two cups of cooked quinoa, chilled
- 1 cup frozen chopped spinach, thawed
- 1 pound 93%-lean ground turkey
- ½ cup crumbled feta cheese
- 2 tbsp lemon juice
- 2 cups sliced cucumber
- 1-pint cherry tomatoes
- ¼ cup tzatziki
- 1 tbsp olive oil
- half cup parsley chopped
- 3 tbsp chopped mint

Instructions

You need to follow the under mentioned instructions for preparing this Mediterranean breakfast recipe:

1. Squeeze the spinach to remove any excess moisture. In a medium mixing bowl, combine spinach, feta, turkey, 1/8 tsp salt, garlic powder, oregano and 1/8 teaspoon pepper. Make 12 meatballs out of the mixture, over medium heat, heat a big nonstick skillet. Spray the pan with the cooking spray. Add meatballs to the pan, working in batches if necessary. Then cook till browned on all sides and no more pink in the center, approximately 10 to 12 minutes. (If you stick an instant-read thermometer in the center, it should read 165 degrees F.) Allow the meatballs to cool before serving.

2. In a medium mixing bowl, combine the lemon juice, oil, quinoa, parsley, mint and the remaining 1/4 tsp salt and pepper. Divide the mixture between four single-serving lidded containers. Take three meatballs, 1/2 cup cucumbers, and 1/2 cup cherry tomatoes and put them on top of each.

3. Refrigerate for a maximum of 4 days after sealing the containers. Refrigerate the tzatziki in four small containers.

4. Move the meatballs to a microwave-safe container. Do not forget to heat till steaming before serving. Serve with tzatziki.

2. Mason jar power salad with Chickpeas & Tuna

Preparation time

5 minutes

Servings

1 person

Nutritional facts

430 calories

Ingredients

We have listed below the ingredients that are required for making this breakfast recipe:

- 3 cups chopped kale bite-size pieces
- ½ cup rinsed canned chickpeas
- 2 tbsp vinaigrette (honey-mustard)
- one 2.5-ounces pouched tuna in the water
- one carrot, peeled & shredded

Instructions

You need to follow the under mentioned instructions for preparing this Mediterranean breakfast recipe:

1. In a bowl, toss the kale with the dressing, then transfer to a one-quarter mason jar. Tuna, chickpeas, & carrots go on top. Refrigerate for a maximum of two days after screwing the lid on the jar.
2. For serving, empty the contents of the jar into a mixing bowl & toss with the dressed kale to mix salad ingredients.

3. Mediterranean Chicken with Orzo Salad

Preparation time

40 minutes

Servings

4 persons

Nutritional facts

402 calories

Ingredients

We have listed below the ingredients that are required for making this breakfast recipe:

- ½ teaspoon salt, divided

- half teaspoon ground pepper, evenly divided
- 2 tablespoons lemon juice
- 1 clove garlic, grated
- 2 teaspoons chopped fresh oregano
- ¾ cups of orzo whole-wheat
- 2 cups baby spinach thinly sliced
- 1 cup cucumber chopped
- 2 skinless, boneless chicken breasts (8 ounces each), halved
- 3 tablespoons extra-virgin olive oil, divided
- 1 teaspoon lemon zest
- 1 cup tomato chopped
- ¼ cup of red onion chopped
- ¼ cup feta cheese crumbled
- 2 tablespoons Kalamata olives chopped

Instructions

You need to follow the under mentioned instructions for preparing this Mediterranean breakfast recipe:

1. Preheat the oven to 425 degrees Fahrenheit.
2. Take one tablespoon oil, lemon zest, & 1/4 teaspoon salt & pepper and brush on chicken. Then put in a baking dish, combine all of the ingredients. Bake for 25 to 30 minutes, or till the thermometer instant-read put in thickest part reads 165 degrees F.
3. Meanwhile, in a medium saucepan over high heat, bring a quart of the water to boil. Cook for eight minutes after adding the orzo. Cook for an additional minute after adding the spinach. Rinse with chilled water after draining. Drain well & place in a large mixing bowl. Cucumber, onion, tomato, feta, & olives are all good additions. To combine, stir everything together.
4. In a small bowl, combine the remaining two tbsp of oil, oregano, garlic, lemon juice, and the remaining 1/4 teaspoon salt & pepper. All except one tablespoon of dressing should be incorporated into the orzo mixture. Serve with the salad and remaining dressing drizzled over the chicken.

4. Tomato-&-Avocado Cheese Sandwich
Preparation time

15 minutes

Servings

1 person

Nutritional facts

439 calories

Ingredients

We have listed below the ingredients that are required for making this breakfast recipe:

- 3 slices tomato
- 2 teaspoons balsamic vinegar
- 1 medium ripe pear
- ¼ cup grated Parmesan cheese
- 1 cup mixed salad greens or baby spinach
- 2 slices whole-wheat bread
- ¼ avocado, mashed

Instructions

You need to follow the under mentioned instructions for preparing this Mediterranean breakfast recipe:

1. Place the bread on the work surface. On one slice, spread avocado. Toss in some tomatoes and a sprinkling of cheese. 4 to 6 minutes in a toaster oven, toast both pieces of bread till the plain piece is toasted as well as the cheese on the topped piece is starting to melt.

2. With a spatula, remove the toast from the toaster oven and pile greens or spinach on top of the cheese side. Top with the remainder toast and a drizzle of vinegar. If desired, cut in half and serve with pear.

5. Tomato, Cucumber & White-Bean Salad with Basil Vinaigrette

Preparation time

25 minutes

Servings

4 persons

Nutritional facts

246 calories

Ingredients

We have listed below the ingredients that are required for making this breakfast recipe:

- 1 tablespoon shallot finely chopped

- 2 tsp Dijon mustard
- one (15 ounces) cannellini low-sodium beans can be rinsed
- 1 cup grape or cherry tomatoes halved
- ½ cucumber, cut into halves lengthwise & sliced (one cup)
- 1 teaspoon honey
- ¼ teaspoon salt
- ¼ teaspoon ground pepper
- ½ cup packed fresh basil leaves
- ¼ cup extra-virgin olive oil
- 3 tablespoons red-wine vinegar
- 10 cups mixed salad greens

Instructions

You need to follow the under mentioned instructions for preparing this Mediterranean breakfast recipe:

1. In a mini food processor, combine vinegar, basil, oil, mustard, salt shallot, honey, and pepper. Process until the mixture is mostly smooth.
2. Place in a large mixing bowl. Combine the greens, tomatoes, beans, and cucumber in a large mixing bowl. Toss to evenly coat.

6. Chopped Mediterranean Salad

Preparation time

20 minutes

Servings

2 persons

Nutritional facts

100 calories

Ingredients

We have listed below the ingredients that are required for making this breakfast recipe:

- ⅓ cup chopped seeded tomato
- 1 cup mixed salad greens
- 2 tablespoons crumbled reduced-fat feta cheese
- ⅓ cup chopped zucchini

- ⅓ cup chopped yellow or orange bell pepper
- ⅓ cup very small broccoli florets
- 1 tablespoon purchased basil pesto
- 2 teaspoons white balsamic vinegar or regular balsamic vinegar

Instructions

You need to follow the under mentioned instructions for preparing this Mediterranean breakfast recipe:

1. In a small bowl, combine the pesto and vinegar. Combine the tomato, zucchini, bell pepper, and broccoli in a mixing bowl.
2. Divide the greens between two serving plates if desired. Serve with the vegetable mixture on top. Feta cheese should be sprinkled on top.

7. Grilled Vegetable Salads with Goat Cheese

Preparation time

10 minutes

Servings

4 persons

Nutritional facts

347 calories

Ingredients

We have listed below the ingredients that are required for making this breakfast recipe:

- ¼ cup unsalted roasted sunflower seeds
- 1/2 cup balsamic & fig dressing
- 1package (10 ounces) Tuscan kale
- 4 ounces herb-coated or marinated goat cheese
- 1 package(16 ounces) grilled vegetables frozen and marinated

Instructions

You need to follow the under mentioned instructions for preparing this Mediterranean breakfast recipe:

1. Divide the kale evenly between four one-serving lidded boxes. Put one ounce of goat cheese & 1 tbsp sunflower seeds on top of each. Refrigerate for a maximum of 4 days after sealing the containers.

2. Refrigerate two tsp dressing in each of four tiny lidded containers for up to four days.

3. Transfer one-quarter of grilled vegetables (approximately one cup) to any of the meal-preparing boxes the night before you take your lunch to go; frozen vegetables would be thawed & ready to be eaten by lunchtime, just before serving drizzle salad with the dressing.

8. Pasta, Tuna & Roasted Pepper Salad

Preparation time

30 minutes

Servings

4 persons

Nutritional facts

258 calories

Ingredients

We have listed below the ingredients that are required for making this breakfast recipe:

- half cup scallions or red onion, finely chopped
- 2 tbsp capers, rinsed, finely chopped if big
- 2 tbsp plain yogurt, nonfat
- ⅛ teaspoon salt, or to taste
- Freshly ground pepper, to taste
- 6 ounces whole-wheat penne or rigatoni (1 3/4 cups)
- 2 tbsp fresh basil, chopped
- 1 6-ounce can chunk light tuna in water, drained
- 1 7-ounce jar roasted red peppers, rinsed and sliced (2/3 cup), divided
- 1 tbsp olive oil extra-virgin
- 1 ½ tsp lemon juice
- 1 tiny clove of garlic, crushed & peeled

Instructions

You need to follow the under mentioned instructions for preparing this Mediterranean breakfast recipe:

1. To begin, bring a big pot of salted water to a boil.

2. In a large mixing bowl, mix tuna, one-third cup of red peppers, scallions or onion & capers.

3. In a blender or food processor, combine the basil, oil, yogurt, lemon juice, salt, garlic, pepper, and remaining one-third cup red peppers. Puree until completely smooth.

4. Cook pasta for 10-14 mins, or as directions on the package, until just tender. Drain & rinse thoroughly with cold water. Toss in with tuna mixture and red pepper sauce to coat.

9. Five Minute Mediterranean Bowl-Healthy Lunch Meal Prep Recipe

Preparation time

10 minutes

Servings

2 persons

Nutritional facts

174 calories

Ingredients

We have listed below the ingredients that are required for making this lunch recipe:

- a tiny bunch of chopped parsley,
- 2-3 tbsp quinoa, cooked
- black pepper, freshly ground
- 1 or 2 spring onions, finely chopped
- some olive oil
- 7 to 8 olives
- one-third cup of canned chickpeas, rinsed and drained
- one tbsp tzatziki
- 1 small cucumber, cubed
- Half cup cherry tomatoes halved
- Two tablespoons hummus

Instructions

You need to follow the under mentioned instructions for preparing this Mediterranean lunch recipe:

1. Clean and cut the vegetables and put them in a mixing bowl. To taste, apply vinegar, olive oil and salt.

2. Assemble the bowl. Salad, chickpeas that have been rinsed and washed, olives, quinoa. Two tbsp hummus and one tablespoon tzatziki along with freshly ground black pepper in the center / on top. It is ready.

10. Mediterranean Bento Lunch

Preparation time

15 minutes

Servings

1 person

Nutritional facts

497 calories

Ingredients

We have listed below the ingredients that are required for making this lunch recipe:

- Quarter cup diced tomato
- One tbsp diced olives
- One tbsp crumbled feta cheese
- One cup grapes
- Quarter cup chickpeas, rinsed
- Quarter cup diced cucumber
- 1 whole-wheat pita bread, quartered
- Two tbsp hummus
- One tbsp chopped fresh parsley
- half teaspoon extra-virgin olive oil
- One tsp red-wine vinegar
- 3 ounces grilled turkey breast tenderloin or chicken breast

Instructions

You need to follow the under mentioned instructions for preparing this Mediterranean lunch recipe:

- In a medium bowl, toss the chickpeas, cucumber, onion, parsley, olives, feta, oil and vinegar together. Pack it in a medium-sized jar.
- In a medium container, put the turkey (or chicken).
- In small packets, pack grapes and pita and hummus in a dip-size container.

11. Greek Chicken & Cucumber Pita Sandwiches with Yogurt Sauce

Preparation time

1 hour 45 minutes

Servings

4 persons

Nutritional facts

353 calories

Ingredients

We have listed below the ingredients that are required for making this lunch recipe:

- One tbsp freshly chopped oregano or One tsp dried
- two ¾ teaspoons garlic, minced divided
- half cup sliced red onion
- One cup chopped plum tomatoes
- ¼ teaspoon red pepper crushed
- chicken tenders 1 pound
- one English cucumber, cut into halves, seeded & grated, also half English cucumber, sliced
- half tsp salt, divided
- Greek yogurt ¾ cup nonfat and plain
- two tsp fresh mint chopped
- One tsp lemon zest
- Two tbsp fresh lemon juice
- 5 teaspoons olive oil, divided
- two teaspoons fresh dill chopped
- One tsp ground pepper
- two (6 1/2 inches) pita bread (whole-wheat), halved
- four lettuce leaves

Instructions

You need to follow the under mentioned instructions for preparing this Mediterranean lunch recipe:

1. Mix lemon juice, three tsp oil, lemon zest oregano, two teaspoons garlic in a large bowl along with crushed red pepper. Insert the chicken and coat with a toss. Marinate for a minimum of 1 hr or up to 4 hrs in the refrigerator.

2. Meanwhile, toss with a quarter tsp of salt the grated cucumber. Leave for 15 mins to drain. Then press to release extra liquid. then Transfer to a medium bowl. Combine the yogurt, dill, mint, ground pepper & the other 2 tsp of oil, 3/4 teaspoon Garlic, and a quarter teaspoon of salt. To serve, refrigerate until it is ready.

3. Preheat a grill to mid-high temperature.

4. Oil the rack for the grill. Grill chicken until 165 degrees F is registered by an automatic thermometer put in the middle.

5. Spread some sauce within each half of the pita for serving. Insert the chicken, the lettuce, the red onion, the tomatoes and the cucumber that has been cut into slices.

12. Prosciutto, Mozzarella & Melon Plate

Preparation time

20 minutes

Servings

2 persons

Nutritional facts

546 calories

Ingredients

We have listed below the ingredients that are required for making this lunch recipe:

- 6 thin slices of prosciutto, cut in half
- half cup unsalted hazelnuts
- 4 chocolate-dipped strawberries
- 10 small fresh mozzarella balls
- half cup cherry tomato halves
- One cupcubed cantaloupe
- 6 (1/4 inch thick) slices whole-wheat baguette

Instructions

You need to follow the under mentioned instructions for preparing this Mediterranean lunch recipe:

1. Divide items equally between two plates.

13. Mediterranean Lentil & Kale Salad

Preparation time

15 minutes

Servings

4 persons

Nutritional facts

186 calories

Ingredients

We have listed below the ingredients that are required for making this lunch recipe:

- One tbsp finely chopped dried tomatoes (not oil-packed)
- Quarter cup shredded Parmesan cheese (1/2 ounce)
- 1 clove garlic, minced
- half teaspoon Dijon-style mustard
- ¼ teaspoon salt
- ¼ teaspoon black pepper
- 1 ounce 1 5-ounce package (8 cups) fresh baby kale
- 1 ounce 1 9-ounce package refrigerated steamed lentils, such as Melissa's®
- Quarter cup red wine vinegar
- Two tbsp olive oil
- One cup chopped red sweet pepper

Instructions

You need to follow the under mentioned instructions for preparing this Mediterranean lunch recipe:

1. For the vinaigrette, mix together the olive oil, red wine vinegar, chopped tomatoes, salt, garlic, mustard and pepper in a wide serving bowl.
2. Insert kale; coat with a toss. Top with sweet pepper and lentils and sprinkle the cheese.

CHAPTER 5: Mediterranean Diet Dinner Recipes

Make healthy and delicious Mediterranean diet dinner recipes and enjoy a healthy and satisfying life.

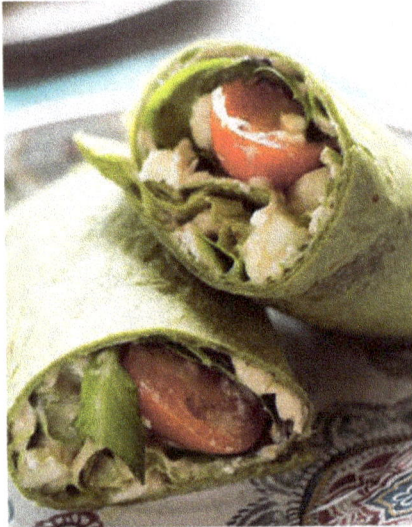

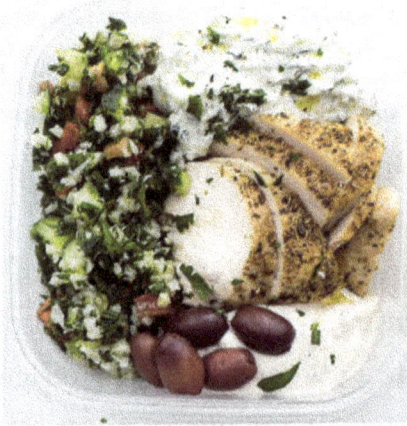

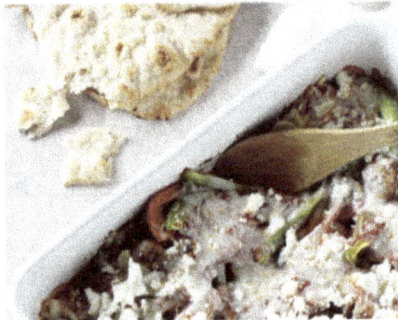

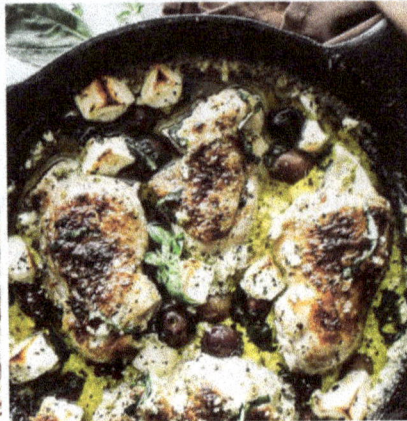

1. Traditional Greek Salad

Preparation time

30 minutes

Servings

4 persons

Nutritional facts

102.9 calories

Ingredients

We have listed below the ingredients that are required for making this dinner recipe:

- 1 English cucumber (hothouse cucumber) partially peeled, making a striped pattern
- 1 green bell pepper cored
- 1/Two tablespoons dried oregano
- Greek pitted Kalamata olives a handful to your liking
- kosher salt a pinch
- 1 medium red onion
- 4 Medium juicy tomatoes
- 4 tbsp quality extra virgin olive oil
- 1-Two tablespoons red wine vinegar
- Blocks of Greek feta cheese do not crumble the feta. Leave it in large pieces

Instructions

You need to follow the under mentioned instructions for preparing this Mediterranean dinner recipe:

1. Slice the red onion in half and slice thinly into half-moons. (Before adding to the salad, put the sliced onions in a solution of iced water and vinegar for a while if you want to take the edge off.
2. Cut the tomatoes into wedges or big pieces.
3. The partly peeled cucumber is sliced in half lengthwise and cut into thick halves (at least 1/2" thick)
4. Cut the bell pepper thinly into rings.
5. Place it all in a big salad bowl. Insert a healthy handful of pitted olives into the kalamata.
6. Season with kosher salt very finely (just a pinch) and a touch of dried oregano.
7. Pour all over the salad olive oil and red wine vinegar. Give it all a really soft toss to blend.
8. Now add the top of the feta blocks and add a little more dried oregano.
9. Serve with bread that is crusty.

2. Mediterranean Watermelon Salad Recipe

Preparation time

30 minutes

Servings

4 persons

Nutritional facts

192 calories

Ingredients

We have listed below the ingredients that are required for making this dinner recipe:

- 1 to Two tablespoons quality extra virgin olive oil
- pinch of salt
- 15 fresh basil leaves, chopped
- Half cup crumbled feta cheese, more to your liking
- 1/2 watermelon, peeled, cut into cubes
- 1 English (or Hot House) cucumber, cubed (about 2 cupfuls of cubed cucumbers)
- Two tablespoons honey
- Two tablespoons lime juice
- 15 fresh mint leaves, chopped

Instructions

You need to follow the under mentioned instructions for preparing this Mediterranean dinner recipe:

1. Whisk the lime juice, honey, olive oil and a sprinkle of salt together in a small bowl. Set aside.
2. The cucumbers, watermelon and fresh herbs are mixed in a large bowl.
3. Top with the honey vinaigrette the watermelon salad and gently toss to blend. Put the feta cheese on top and serve.

3. Tabouli Salad Recipe (Tabbouleh)

Preparation time

20 minutes

Servings

4 persons

Nutritional facts

190 calories

Ingredients

We have listed below the ingredients that are required for making this dinner recipe:

- one English cucumber or hothouse cucumber, finely chopped
- two bunches of parsley stems removed, rinsed and dried, finely chopped

- Romaine lettuce leaves to serve, optional
- 12 to 15 mint leaves (fresh), stems removed, rinsed, dried, finely chopped
- four green onions, green and white parts, finely diced
- Salt
- Half cup extra fine bulgur wheat
- 4 firm Roma tomatoes, very finely chopped
- 3 to 4 tbsp of lime juice or lemon juice
- 3 to 4 tbsp of extra virgin Early Harvest olive oil

Instructions

You need to follow the under mentioned instructions for preparing this Mediterranean dinner recipe:

1. Wash and soak Bulgur wheat in the water for 5 to 7 minutes. Drain well. Remove any extra water by squeezing with hands. And put aside.
2. The vegetables, green onions and herbs are very finely chopped. To drain the excess juice, make sure to put tomatoes in a colander.
3. In a mixing bowl or dish, put the diced vegetables, green onion and herbs. Add bulgur and use salt for seasoning. Gently mix.
4. Lime juice & olive oil can now be applied and combined again.
5. Cover the tabouli for the best results, then refrigerate for thirty minutes. Move to a dish for serving. Serve tabouli with a side of leaves of romaine lettuce and pita if you like, which serve as wraps for tabouli or 'boats.'
6. Hummus, Roasted Hummus of Red Pepper or Baba Ganoush are other appetizers to serve next to tabouli salad.

4. Greek Lemon Rice Recipe

Preparation time

45 minutes

Servings

4 persons

Nutritional facts

145 calories

Ingredients

We have listed below the ingredients that are required for making this dinner recipe:

- 1 medium-sized yellow onion, diced (just over One cup chopped onions)

- Large handful chopped fresh parsley
- 1 tsp dill weed (dry dill)
- 1 minced garlic clove,
- Half cup orzo pasta
- two juice lemons (and 1 lemon zest)
- two cups broth low sodium(vegetable or chicken broth would work)
- a Pinch of salt
- two cups long grain rice (uncooked)
- Early Harvest Greek extra virgin olive oil

Instructions

You need to follow the under mentioned instructions for preparing this Mediterranean dinner recipe:

1. Wash the rice well and then soak it in a lot of cold water for around 15 to 20 minutes (enough to cover the rice by 1 inch). By merely putting it between your thumb and index finger, you should be able to split a grain of rice quickly. Drain perfect.

2. In a wide saucepan with a lid, heat about 3 tbsp extra virgin olive oil until the oil shimmers but does not smoke. Insert the onions and cook until translucent, around 3 to 4 minutes. Add the orzo pasta and garlic. Toss about until the orzo has acquired some color, and then stir in the rice for a little while. Toss to coat.

3. Insert lemon juice and broth now. Get the liquid (it should decrease a little) to a rolling boil, then turn the heat off. Cover and cook for 20 minutes or until the rice is ready.

4. Remove the rice from the heat. Keep it covered for the best results, and do not mess with rice for another 10 minutes or so.

5. Uncover and mix parsley, dill weed and lemon zest and stir. Put a handful of slices of lemon on top for garnish, if you prefer. Enjoy.

5. Mediterranean Quinoa Bowls with Roasted Red Pepper Sauce
Preparation time

20 minutes

Servings

1person

Nutritional facts

381 calories

Ingredients

We have listed below the ingredients that are required for making this breakfast recipe:

- juice of one lemon
- thinly sliced red onion
- hummus
- fresh basil or parsley
- olive oil, lemon juice, salt, pepper
- 1/2 cup olive oil
- 1/2 cup almonds
- cooked quinoa
- 1 16 ounces jar roasted red peppers, drained
- 1 clove garlic
- 1/2 teaspoon salt (more to taste)
- spinach, kale, or cucumber
- feta cheese
- kalamata olives
- pepperoncini

Instructions

You need to follow the under mentioned instructions for preparing this Mediterranean breakfast recipe:

1. In a food processor or blender, pulse all of the sauce ingredients until they are mostly smooth. The texture should be textured and thick.
2. Cook the quinoa as directed on the package. Build a Mediterranean Quinoa Bowl once the quinoa is done.
3. Keep leftovers in separate containers as well as assemble each bowl well before serving, particularly the greens and sauces, which will become soggy if stored with the rest of the ingredients.

6. Baked Chicken and Ricotta Meatballs

Preparation time

35 minutes

Servings

4 persons

Nutritional facts

454 calories

Ingredients

We have listed below the ingredients that are required for making this breakfast recipe:

- Kosher salt and freshly ground black pepper
- 1 pound ground chicken, preferably dark meat
- Juice of 1 lemon
- Grated Parmesan for sprinkling
- ½ teaspoon crushed red pepper flakes, or more if desired
- 1 large egg
- 2 garlic cloves, grated
- ¾ cup ricotta cheese, drained and lightly salted
- ½ cup parsley leaves and fine stems, roughly chopped
- 14 ounces (400g) broccolini, rough stems trimmed and thick pieces cut lengthwise
- 1 lemon, ends trimmed and thinly sliced
- 4 tablespoons extra-virgin olive oil, divided
- ¾ cup panko breadcrumbs

Instructions

You need to follow the under mentioned instructions for preparing this Mediterranean breakfast recipe:

1. Preheat the oven to 425 degrees Fahrenheit.
2. Put the broccoli as well as lemon slices with three tbsp olive oil, salt, pepper, and red pepper flakes on a baking sheet. While preparing the meatballs, evenly spread on the baking sheet as well as set aside.
3. In a medium mixing bowl, whisk together the egg, garlic, ricotta, one teaspoon salt, parsley, pepper, the remaining oil, breadcrumbs, and meat with your hands. Remember that too much mushing will make them tough and dry. Through the seasonings, you should still be able to see pieces of meat. Using a gentle rolling motion between your hands, lightly wet the hands with water and/or oil. Then roll the meat into 20 loose—not tightly packed—rounds, relatively smaller than golf balls. Remember that the water will keep them from sticking to your hands. To make cleanup easier, place large pieces of baking parchment on the counter.

4. Place the meatballs between the broccoli as well as lemon on the baking sheet. Bake for 15 to 20 minutes, or when the meatballs are browned as well as cooked through, and the broccoli is crisp, shaking the baking sheet to move the meatballs and rotating the tray halfway through to ensure even cooking.

5. Remove from the oven, drizzle with lemon juice, and divide among plates. If using, top with grated Parmesan.

7. Mediterranean Couscous with Tuna and Pepperoncini

Preparation time

15 minutes

Servings

4 persons

Nutritional facts

226 calories

Ingredients

We have listed below the ingredients that are required for making this breakfast recipe:

- Two cans oil tuna of 5-ounce
- Extra-virgin olive oil, for serving
- Kosher salt and freshly ground black pepper
- 1 lemon, quartered
- one pint of cherry tomatoes, cut into halves
- half cup sliced pepperoncini
- ⅓ cup fresh parsley chopped
- 1 cup chicken broth or water
- 1¼ cups couscous
- ¾ teaspoon kosher salt
- ¼ cup capers

Instructions

You need to follow the under mentioned instructions for preparing this Mediterranean breakfast recipe:

1. Bring broth and/or the water to boil in a small pot over medium-high heat. Turn off the heat, then stir in couscous, & cover the pot. Allow for a 10-minute rest period.

2. Meanwhile, combine the tomatoes, pepperoni, tuna, parsley & capers in a medium mixing bowl.

3. Season with pepper and salt & drizzle with some olive oil after fluffing couscous with a fork. Serve with the lemon wedges on top of the couscous and tuna mixture.

8. Balsamic One Pan Chicken and Veggies

Preparation time

30 minutes

Servings

4 persons

Nutritional facts

383.51 calories

Ingredients

We have listed below the ingredients that are required for making this breakfast recipe:

- 1 bunch asparagus (trimmed and cut into bite-sized pieces)
- ½ zucchini (cut into bite-sized pieces)
- ¼ teaspoon salt
- ½ cup feta cheese crumbled
- ¼ cup pomegranate arils
- 1 tablespoon arrowroot starch (corn starch or all-purpose flour may be used)
- one lb skinless, boneless chicken breast (almost 2 big chicken breasts; cut into 1-inch cubes)
- 1 cup chicken stock
- two tbsp olive oil (divided)
- 3 cups baby potatoes (quartered)
- salt and pepper
- ¼ cup balsamic vinegar

Instructions

You need to follow the under mentioned instructions for preparing this Mediterranean breakfast recipe:

1. In a large skillet, heat one tablespoon of oil over medium heat.
2. Season with salt and pepper and add the potatoes. Cook, covered, until fork-tender, about 30 minutes (roughly 15 minutes).
3. Toss in the asparagus and zucchini, stir well, cover, as well as cook for five minutes, stirring once.

4. Sprinkle arrowroot starch over the potatoes, asparagus, and zucchini in a large mixing bowl. Set aside after tossing to coat.

5. Cook for 7-10 minutes, until the chicken, is cooked through, in the pan with the remaining one tbsp of olive oil.

6. Return the vegetables, chicken stock, balsamic vinegar, and salt to the pan. Cook for 3-5 minutes, occasionally stirring, till the sauce bubbles as well as thickens.

7. Serve immediately with pomegranates and feta cheese.

9. One-Skillet Greek Sun-Dried Tomato Chicken And Farro

Preparation time

55 minutes

Servings

6 persons

Nutritional facts

366 calories

Ingredients

We have listed below the ingredients that are required for making this breakfast recipe:

- 2 tablespoons balsamic vinegar
- 1 tablespoon chopped fresh dill
- 8 ounces feta cheese, cubed
- 1 tablespoon chopped fresh dill
- 3 tablespoons toasted pine nuts
- 1 tablespoon chopped fresh oregano
- 1 tablespoon paprika
- 2 cloves garlic, minced or grated
- 2 tablespoons extra virgin olive oil
- 1 pound boneless, skinless chicken breasts, or small thighs
- 1/4 cup extra virgin olive oil
- kosher salt and black pepper
- 1 cup uncooked farro or quinoa
- 2 1/2 cups low sodium chicken broth
- 2 cups baby spinach
- 1/2 cup oil-packed sun-dried tomatoes

- 1/3 cup kalamata olives, pitted
- juice of 1 lemon

Instructions

You need to follow the under mentioned instructions for preparing this Mediterranean breakfast recipe:

1. Preheat oven to 400 degrees Fahrenheit.
2. Mix two tbsp olive oil, dill, chicken, oregano, balsamic garlic vinegar, paprika, and a large pinch of salt & pepper in a medium mixing bowl. Toss well to coat the chicken evenly.
3. In a cast-iron skillet, heat the remaining 2 tablespoons olive oil over medium-high heat. When the oil is hot, add the chicken and cook until golden brown on both sides, approximately 3-5 minutes per side. Take the chicken out of the skillet and set it aside.
4. Add the farro to the same skillet. Cook for 2-3 mins. Add the olives, spinach, sun-dried tomatoes and lemon juice to the chicken broth. Bring to a boil over high heat, stirring constantly. Return the chicken to the skillet, along with any juices left on the plate. Transfer to the oven and roast for twenty minutes, or until the chicken is fully cooked and the farro has softened.
5. Serve the chicken with feta cheese, dill and pine nuts on top.

10. Lemon Salmon with Garlic and Thyme

Preparation time

25 minutes

Servings

4 persons

Nutritional facts

356 calories

Ingredients

We have listed below the ingredients that are required for making this breakfast recipe:

- Kosher salt and freshly ground black pepper
- ½ teaspoon dried thyme
- 4 to 5 five garlic cloves, peeled and lightly crushed

- 1 whole lemon, zested and sliced into thin rounds
- Four 5- to 6-ounce salmon fillets
- Extra virgin olive oil, as needed

Instructions

You need to follow the under mentioned instructions for preparing this Mediterranean breakfast recipe:

1. Preheat the oven to 400 degrees Fahrenheit.
2. Drizzle a little olive oil over the salmon fillets in a baking dish. Add salt and pepper, then top with lemon zest and thyme evenly. Add the garlic cloves to the dish after placing the lemon slices on top of the fillets.
3. Bake for 18-20 minutes, or until the salmon is cooked through and flakes easily with a fork. Remember to adjust the baking time if the fillets are very thick or thin.

11. Chickpea Vegetable Coconut Curry

Preparation time

30 minutes

Servings

4 persons

Nutritional facts

665 calorics

Ingredients

We have listed below the ingredients that are required for making this breakfast recipe:

- 3 garlic cloves, minced
- 1 small head cauliflower, cut into bite-size florets
- 2 teaspoons chili powder
- Kosher salt and freshly ground black pepper
- Steamed rice, for serving
- ¼ cup chopped fresh cilantro
- 4 scallions, thinly sliced
- 1 teaspoon ground coriander
- 1 tablespoon extra-virgin olive oil
- 1 red onion, thinly sliced
- 1 red bell pepper, thinly sliced

- 1 tablespoon fresh ginger, minced
- 3 tablespoons red curry paste
- One 14-ounce can of coconut milk
- 1 lime, halved
- One 28-ounce can of chickpeas
- 1½ cups frozen peas

Instructions

You need to follow the under mentioned instructions for preparing this Mediterranean breakfast recipe:

1. Heat the olive oil in a large saucepan over medium heat. Cook, occasionally stirring, until the onion and bell pepper are almost tender, approximately 5 minutes. Insert the garlic and ginger and cook for 1 minute, or until fragrant.

2. Toss in the cauliflower until everything is well combined. Cook, constantly stirring, until the chili powder, coriander, and red curry paste begins to caramelize, approximately 1 minute.

3. Over medium-low heat, stir in the coconut milk as well as bring the mixture to a simmer. Cover the saucepan as well as continue to cook for another 8 to 10 minutes, just until the cauliflower is tender.

4. Remove the lid and stir in the lime juice until everything is well combined. Return the mixture to a simmer, season with salt and pepper, and add the chickpeas and peas.

5. If desired, serve with rice. One tbsp cilantro and 1 tablespoon scallions should be garnished on each serving.

12. Easy Greek-Style Eggplant Recipe

Preparation time

1 hour 15 minutes

Servings

4 persons

Nutritional facts

240 calories

Ingredients

We have listed below the ingredients that are required for making this dinner recipe:

- Extra Virgin Olive Oil
- 1 large yellow onion, chopped
- 1 28-oz can chopped tomato
- 2 15-oz cans chickpeas, reserve the canning liquid
- Fresh herbs such as parsley and mint for garnish
- 1 green bell pepper, stem and innards removed, diced
- 1 carrot, chopped
- 6 large garlic cloves, minced
- 2 dry bay leaves
- 1 to 1 ½ tsp sweet paprika OR smoked paprika
- 1.5 lb eggplant, cut into cubes
- Kosher salt
- 1 tsp organic ground coriander
- 1 tsp dry oregano
- ¾ tsp ground cinnamon
- ½ tsp organic ground turmeric
- ½ tsp black pepper

Instructions

You need to follow the under mentioned instructions for preparing this Mediterranean dinner recipe:

1. Heat the oven to 400 degrees F.
2. Place eggplant cubes over a wide bowl or directly over your sink in a colander, and sprinkle them with salt. Put aside for 20 minutes or so to encourage some bitterness to "sweat out" the eggplant. Use water to clean and pat dry.
3. Heat quarter cup extra virgin olive oil at medium-high in a large braiser until shimmering but not burning. Add the chopped onions, peppers, and carrot. Cook, constantly stirring, for 2-3 minutes, then add the garlic, bay leaf, spices, and a splash of salt. Cook for another minute, until fragrant, stirring.
4. Eggplant, sliced tomatoes, chickpeas and reserved chickpea liquid are now added. Stir to blend.
5. Carry it to a rolling boil for about 10 minutes. Stir regularly. Remove, cover and switch to the oven from the stovetop.
6. Heat in the oven for 45 minutes until the eggplant is completely cooked. (While braising eggplant, be sure to inspect once or twice and see whether there is a need

for more liquid. If so, momentarily remove from the oven and stir in around half a cup of water at a time.

7. Remove from the oven when the eggplant is ready and apply a generous drizzle of Private Reserve EVOO and garnish with fresh herbs (parsley or mint). A side of Greek yogurt or even pita bread or Tzatziki sauce is served hot or at room temperature.

13. Baked Lemon Garlic Salmon Recipe

Preparation time

28 minutes

Servings

4 persons

Nutritional facts

388 calories

Ingredients

We have listed below the ingredients that are required for making this dinner recipe:

- olive oil Extra virgin
- 1/2 lemon, cut into rounds
- 2 tsp dry oregano
- 1 tsp sweet paprika
- 1/2 tsp black pepper
- Parsley
- one large lemon (Zest)
- Juice of two lemons
- 2 lb salmon fillet
- Kosher salt
- 3 tbsp olive oil extra virgin
- 5 chopped garlic cloves,

Instructions

You need to follow the under mentioned instructions for preparing this Mediterranean dinner recipe:

1. Preheat oven to 375 degrees F.

2. Prepare a sauce consisting of lemon garlic. Mix the olive oil extra virgin, lemon juice, lemon zest, oregano, garlic, black pepper and paprika together in a small bowl or measuring cup. Give a nice whisk to the sauce.

3. Prepare a sheet pan with a big foil piece lined with. Brush the olive oil on top of the foil.

4. Dry pat salmon now and season with kosher salt on both sides well. Put it on a sheet of foiled paper. Top with sauce of lemon garlic (ensure to spread sauce evenly.)

5. Then Fold film over salmon. Bake for 15-20 mins until the thickest portion of the salmon's almost fully cooked through (cooking time may differ depending on the fish's thickness. If the salmon is smaller, check various minutes early to make sure that the salmon doesn't overcook. It can take a little longer if your slice is quite thick, 1 1/2 inches. or more)

6. To uncover the top of the salmon, gently remove it from the oven and open the foil. Place it momentarily, around 3 mins or so, under the broiler. To ensure it does not overcook & garlic doesn't roast, watch carefully as it broils.

14. Learn to Make Falafel

Preparation time

50 minutes

Servings

2 persons

Nutritional facts

274 calories

Ingredients

We have listed below the ingredients that are required for making this dinner recipe:

- ¾ cup fresh cilantro leaves stem removed
- half cup fresh dill stems removed
- 1 small onion, quartered
- 7-8 garlic cloves, peeled
- English cucumbers, chopped or diced
- Tomatoes, chopped or diced
- Baby Arugula
- Pickles
- Salt to taste

- 1 tbsp ground black pepper
- 1 tbsp ground cumin
- 1 tbsp ground coriander
- two cups dried chickpeas (Do NOT use canned or cooked chickpeas)
- ½ tsp baking soda
- One cup fresh parsley leaves stem removed
- 1 tsp cayenne pepper, optional
- 1 tsp baking powder
- Two tablespoons toasted sesame seeds
- Oil for frying
- Pita pockets

Instructions

You need to follow the under mentioned instructions for preparing this Mediterranean dinner recipe:

1. Put the baking soda and dried chickpeas in a large water-filled bowl to cover at least 2 inches of the chickpeas. Soak for 18 hours overnight. Drain the chickpeas fully when ready and pat them dry.

2. To the large bowl of a food processor equipped with a blade, add the onions, chickpeas, herbs, garlic and spices. Run the food processor for 40 seconds at a time before all of the falafel mixtures are well mixed.

3. Move the falafel mixture into a container and firmly cover it. Refrigerate, until ready to cook, for at least 1 hour or (up to one whole night).

4. Insert the sesame seeds and baking powder into the falafel mixture only prior to frying and swirl with a spoon.

5. Scoop tablespoonfuls of the mixture of falafel and shape them into patties (each 1/2 inch thick). When you shape the patties, it helps to have moist hands.

6. Fill with 3 inches of oil in a medium saucepan. Heat at medium-high until it gently bubbles. Drop the falafel patties carefully in the oil and let them fry for around 3 to 5 minutes or so until the outside is crispy and medium brown. Prevent crowding the falafel in the saucepan. If possible, cook them in batches.

7. Place the fried falafel patties lined with paper towels in a colander or plate to drain.

8. Serve the falafel hot; or place the falafel patties with arugula, tahini or hummus tomato and cucumber in pita bread.

15. Easy Baked Fish with Garlic and Basil

Preparation time

25 minutes

Servings

4 persons

Nutritional facts

280 calories

Ingredients

We have listed below the ingredients that are required for making this dinner recipe:

- 1 1/2 tsp dry oregano
- 1 tsp ground coriander
- 2 bell peppers any color, sliced
- 2 shallots, peeled and sliced
- 1 tsp sweet paprika
- 10 garlic cloves, minced
- 15 basil leaves, sliced into ribbons
- 2 lb fish fillet like halibut
- Salt and pepper
- 6 tbsp extra virgin olive oil
- Juice of 1 lemon

Instructions

You need to follow the under mentioned instructions for preparing this Mediterranean dinner recipe:

1. Dry the fish fillet. Then season with pepper and salt on both sides.
2. Place the fish in a large bag with a zip-top. Insert the paprika, oregano, coriander, minced garlic, spinach, lemon juice and extra virgin olive oil. To ensure that the fish is evenly covered in the marinade, zip the bag shut and massage it. Marinate in the fridge for up to 30 minutes or up to 1 hour.
3. Heat the oven to 425 degrees F.
4. Arrange in the bottom of a 9 by13 baking dish the bell peppers and shallots. Put the fish on top and pour over it the marinade.
5. Bake for 15 minutes or until the fish is finished and flakes easily.

16. Easy Homemade Chicken Shawarma

Preparation time

40 minutes

Servings

4 persons

Nutritional facts

320 calories

Ingredients

We have listed below the ingredients that are required for making this dinner recipe:

- 3/4 tbsp ground coriander
- 3/4 tbsp garlic powder
- Baby arugula
- 3-ingredient Mediterranean Salad
- Pickles or kalamata olives (optional)
- 3/4 tbsp paprika
- 1/2 tsp ground cloves
- 1/2 tsp cayenne pepper, more if you prefer
- Salt
- 8 boneless, skinless chicken thighs
- 1 large onion, thinly sliced
- 3/4 tbsp ground cumin
- 3/4 tbsp turmeric powder
- 1 large lemon, juice of
- 1/3 cup Private Reserve extra virgin olive oil
- 6 pita pockets
- Tahini sauce or Greek Tzatziki sauce

Instructions

You need to follow the under mentioned instructions for preparing this Mediterranean dinner recipe:

1. The cumin, turmeric, coriander, garlic powder, sweet paprika and cloves are mixed in a small bowl. For now, set aside the Shawarma spice mix.

2. Dry the chicken thighs and season on both sides with salt, then thinly slice into tiny bite-sized pieces.

3. The chicken should be put in a large bowl. Insert the spices from the shwarma and toss them to the coat. Add the onions, olive oil, and lemon juice. Again, toss all around. Cover and refrigerate for 3 hours or overnight (you can slash or miss marinating time if you don't have time).

4. Preheat the oven to 425 degrees F when ready. Take the chicken out of the refrigerator and let it sit for a few minutes at room temperature.

5. Spread the marinated chicken on a large lightly-oiled baking sheet pan with the onions in one layer. Roast for 30 minutes in a hot oven at 425 degrees F. Shift the pan to the top rack for a more browned, more crispy chicken and broil very briefly. Take it out of the oven.

6. Prepare the pita pockets as the chicken is roasting. Make tahini sauce. Prepare Mediterranean salad with three ingredients. And put aside.

7. Open up the pita pockets to serve. Insert chicken shawarma, chicken shawarma, arugula, Mediterranean salad and pickles or olives, if you prefer, and scatter some tahini sauce or Tzatziki sauce. Immediately serve.

17. Easy Italian Baked Chicken Recipe

Preparation time

28 minutes

Servings

4 persons

Nutritional facts

290 calories

Ingredients

We have listed below the ingredients that are required for making this dinner recipe:

- 2 tsp/3.6 g dry oregano
- 1 tsp fresh thyme (from 2 springs of thyme)
- Handful chopped fresh parsley for garnish
- Fresh basil leaves for garnish
- 1 tsp/ 2.1 g Sweet paprika
- 4 garlic cloves, minced
- 3 tbsp/ 44.4 ml Extra virgin olive oil
- Juice of 1/2 lemon

- 1 medium red onion, halved and thinly sliced
- 2 lb/907.185 g boneless skinless chicken breast
- Salt and pepper
- 5 to 6 Campari tomatoes (or small Roma tomatoes), halved

Instructions

You need to follow the under mentioned instructions for preparing this Mediterranean dinner recipe:

1. Heat oven to 425 degrees F.
2. Dry chicken. In a large zip-top bag, put a chicken breast and zip the top (make sure to first release some air into the bag), then put it on your poultry cutting board. Pound the chicken to flatten it using a beef mallet. To repeat the procedure with the remaining chicken breast bits, remove them from the zip-top bag and reuse the bag and mallet.
3. Season the chicken on both sides with salt and pepper and put it in a large mixing bowl or dish. Add the spices, extra virgin olive oil, chopped garlic, along with lemon juice. Combine to make sure that the spices and garlic are evenly coated on the chicken.
4. Spread onion slices on the bottom of a big, lightly oiled baking pan. Put the seasoned chicken atop. Then add the tomatoes.
5. The baking dish is to be covered tightly with foil. Then bake for ten minutes while keeping it covered. Then uncover it. Bake for 8 to 10 minutes or so. Be very careful. Depending on the thickness of the chicken breasts, these can require less or more time.
6. Then it should be removed from heat. Let chicken breasts rest for 5 to 10 minutes or so before serving. Uncover and garnish with fresh parsley and basil. Enjoy.

18. Avgolemono Soup Recipe (Greek Lemon Chicken Soup)

Preparation time

35 minutes

Servings

4 persons

Nutritional facts

266 calories

Ingredients

We have listed below the ingredients that are required for making this dinner recipe:

- 1/2 to One cup finely chopped green onions
- 2 garlic cloves, finely chopped
- Half cup freshly-squeezed lemon juice
- 2 large eggs
- Fresh parsley for garnish
- 8 cups low-sodium chicken broth
- 2 bay leaves
- Extra Virgin Olive Oil
- 1/2 to One cup finely chopped carrots
- 1/2 to One cup finely chopped celery
- One cup rice
- Salt and pepper
- 2 cooked boneless chicken breast pieces, shredded

Instructions

You need to follow the under mentioned instructions for preparing this Mediterranean dinner recipe:

1. Heat 1 tbsp olive oil over medium-high heat in a big Dutch oven or heavy pot. Insert the carrots, celery and green onions, briefly toss them together to saute, then stir in the garlic.

2. Insert the chicken broth and bay leaves, and then increase the heat to a high degree. Add the rice, salt and pepper once the liquid comes to a rolling boil. Switch the heat to medium-low and simmer until the rice is tender, or for 20 minutes. Now stir in the chicken that has been cooked.

3. To prepare the egg-lemon sauce, whisk the lemon juice and eggs together in a medium bowl. Insert 2 ladles of the broth from the cooking pot when whisking (this helps temper the eggs). Apply the sauce to the chicken soup until thoroughly mixed and stir. Remove immediately from the heat.

4. Garnish, if you prefer, with fresh parsley. With your favorite bread, serve warm.

19. One-pan Mediterranean Baked Halibut Recipe with Vegetables

Preparation time

25 minutes

Servings

4 persons

Nutritional facts

390 calories

Ingredients

We have listed below the ingredients that are required for making this dinner recipe:

- 1 1/Two tablespoons freshly minced garlic
- two tsp of dill weed
- 1 lb of cherry tomatoes
- one large yellow onion cut into ½ moons
- 1 half lb of halibut fillet, cut into 1 half-inch pieces
- 1 teaspoon seasoned salt
- half tsp black pepper, ground
- 1 teaspoon dried oregano
- Zest of 2 lemons
- Juice of 2 lemons
- One cup Private Reserve Greek extra virgin olive oil
- ¾ to ½ tsp coriander ground
- 1 lb green beans (fresh)

Instructions

You need to follow the under mentioned instructions for preparing this Mediterranean dinner recipe:

1. Heat the oven to 425 degrees F.
2. Whisk ingredients of the sauce together in a big mixing bowl. Insert the tomatoes, green beans, and onions & toss to cover with sauce. Move vegetables to a big baking sheet with a big slotted spatula or spoon (for example, 20 x fifteen x one-inch baking sheets). Put the vegetables on one side of a baking sheet or on 1 half of it and ensure that they're spread in a layer.
3. Now move the strips of halibut fillet to the remaining sauce and toss to cover. To the baking sheet right next to vegetables, move the halibut fillet and add any leftover sauce on the top.
4. Then Lightly sprinkle a little extra seasoned salt with the halibut and vegetables.
5. Bake for 15 minutes in a heated oven at 425 F. Then move baking sheets to the top rack of the oven and broil, watching closely, for another three mins or so. Cherry tomatoes initiate to pop. Underneath the broiler, the cherry tomatoes can begin to pop.

6. Remove baked halibut & vegetables from the oven when ready. It can be served with your preferred Lebanese rice, grain, or pasta. Adding a hearty salad like this Mediterranean Three Bean Salad is a brilliant idea.

20. Easy Homemade Spaghetti Sauce Recipe

Preparation time

35 minutes

Servings

4 persons

Nutritional facts

148 calories

Ingredients

We have listed below the ingredients that are required for making this dinner recipe:

- 2 carrots, finely grated
- 28 oz canned crushed tomatoes
- Handful fresh parsley, about half cup packed, chopped
- 3/4 lb to 1 lb of cooked pasta of your choice
- Half cup water (pasta cooking water, preferred)
- Kosher salt and black pepper
- 1 tbsp dried oregano
- Quarter cup extra virgin olive oil
- 1 medium yellow onion, grated
- 3 garlic cloves, finely minced
- 1 tsp sweet Spanish paprika
- Pinch red pepper flakes, optional
- Handful fresh basil, about half cup, packed, torn

Instructions

You need to follow the under mentioned instructions for preparing this Mediterranean dinner recipe:

1. Heat the extra virgin olive oil on medium heat in a wide pan until it is just shimmering. Add the garlic, onions, and finely grated carrots. Cook for 5 minutes or so, occasionally stirring, until tender.

2. The crushed tomatoes and about half a cup of water are added. A generous pinch of salt and pepper are inserted. Stir in crushed pepper flakes, oregano, paprika if using. Finally, whisk in the parsley and the fresh basil.

3. Bring the sauce to a boil and turn the heat to a low level. Cover it and let it cook for 15 to 20 minutes or so. Check part way, though, and you can add a little more water if you feel the sauce is too thick (some of pasta cooking water). Throw in more fresh basil when the sauce is ready if you prefer.

4. If serving for dinner, add the sauce to the cooked pasta of your preference. Mix to blend and let the pasta cook for around 5 minutes over low heat in the sauce.

21. Greek Chicken Souvlaki Recipe with Tzatziki

Preparation time

4 hours 30 minutes

Servings

4 persons

Nutritional facts

168 calories

Ingredients

We have listed below the ingredients that are required for making this dinner recipe:

- 1 tsp dried rosemary
- Juice of 1 lemon
- 2 bay leaves
- 1 tsp sweet paprika
- 1 tsp each Kosher salt and black pepper
- Quarter cup Private Reserve Greek extra virgin olive oil
- 10 garlic cloves, peeled
- Two tablespoons dried oregano
- Quarter cup dry white wine

Instructions

You need to follow the under mentioned instructions for preparing this Mediterranean dinner recipe:

1. Make the marinade. Insert salt, rosemary, garlic, oregano, paprika, olive oil, pepper, white wine, and lemon juice into the small food processor bowl. Ensure not to add the dried leaves at this stage. Pulse till combined well.

2. In a wide bowl, put the chicken and add the bay leaves. Put the marinade on top. To make sure the chicken is well-coated with marinade, toss to mix. Cover securely and refrigerate overnight or for 2 hours.

3. For 30 to 45 minutes or so, soak 10 to 12 wooden skewers in water. Tzatziki sauce and other fixings are prepared, and if you are using Greek salad or other sides, cook them as well. (It can take longer for certain sides, such as roasted garlic hummus, to prepare them in advance).

4. Thread the marinated chicken parts through the prepared skewers when ready.

5. Set up an outdoor grill (or griddle). With a little oil, brush the grates and heat over medium-high heat. Place chicken skewers on the grill (or cook in batches on the griddle) until well browned and a temperature of 155 ° F is detected on the instant thermometer. To cook on all sides, make sure to turn the skewers uniformly, about 5 minutes in total. (Adjust the grill temperature if necessary). Brush gently with the marinade before grilling (then discard any left marinade).

6. Move the chicken to the serving dish and leave for 3 minutes to rest. Meanwhile, grill the pitas briefly and keep them warm.

7. Assemble grilled pitas for chicken souvlaki. Spread Tzatziki sauce on the pita first, add bits of chicken (take them off skewers first), then add vegetables and olives.

22. Spanakopita Recipe (Greek Spinach Pie)

Preparation time

1 hour 20 minutes

Servings

4 persons

Nutritional facts

393 calories

Ingredients

We have listed below the ingredients that are required for making this dinner recipe:

- 2 minced garlic cloves,

- 1 sixteen oz package of Organic Filo Factory Dough (four pastry sheets), thawed (see tips above)

- One cup Private Reserve olive oil (extra virgin), extra if needed

- Two tablespoons Private Reserve extra virgin olive oil

- 4 eggs

- 10.5 oz quality feta cheese, crumbled

- 2 tsp dried dill weed

- sixteen oz frozen spinach (chopped), thawed and drained
- two bunches parsley,(flat-leaf) stems removed, finely chopped
- one big finely chopped yellow onion,
- black pepper Freshly-ground

Instructions

You need to follow the under mentioned instructions for preparing this Mediterranean dinner recipe:

1. Heat oven to about 325 degrees F.
2. ensure spinach is well drained before you start mixing the filling, & squeeze any extra liquid out by hand.
3. For the filling: Add spinach & remaining ingredients to a mixing bowl. Stir before it is combined.
4. Unroll the sheets of phyllo (fillo) and put them between 2 slightly moist kitchen cloths.
5. Prepare 9 1/2" X 13 inch baking dish. Use olive oil to brush the sides and bottom of the dish.
6. To assemble spanakopita: Put 2 sheets of fillo (phyllo) on the baking dish to cover the sides of the dish. Similarly, apply 2 more sheets and brush with olive oil. Do this again until you have used up two-3rd of phyllo (fillo).
7. Now, scatter the filling of spinach & feta thinly over the fillo(phyllo) crust. Place 2 more sheets on top, and spray with the olive oil.
8. Continue layering the sheets of phyllo (fillo), brushing with olive oil, two at once, until all sheets are used up. Brush with olive oil top layer and spray with only some drops of the water.
9. You can crumble them a little by folding flaps or extra from edges. With olive oil, brush folded edges well. Cut Spanakopita into squares just PART-WAY across, or leave to cut later.
10. Bake for 1 hour in a heated oven at 325 degrees F, till the fillo (phyllo) crust is crispy & golden brown. Take it out of the microwave. Finish cutting and serve in squares. Enjoy, enjoy.

23. Easy Moroccan Vegetable Tagine Recipe

Preparation time

55 minutes

Servings

4 persons

Nutritional facts

448 calories

Ingredients

We have listed below the ingredients that are required for making this dinner recipe:

- 2 large carrots, peeled and chopped
- 2 large russet potatoes, peeled and cubed
- two cups cooked chickpeas
- 1 lemon, juice of
- Handful fresh parsley leaves
- 1 large sweet potato, peeled and cubed
- Salt
- 1 tbsp Harissa spice blend
- 1 tsp ground coriander
- 1 tsp ground cinnamon
- 1/2 tsp ground turmeric
- two cups canned whole peeled tomatoes
- Quarter cup Private Reserve extra virgin olive oil, more for later
- 2 medium yellow onions, peeled and chopped
- 8-10 garlic cloves, peeled and chopped
- Half cup heaping chopped dried apricot
- 1 quart low-sodium vegetable broth (or broth of your choice)

Instructions

You need to follow the under mentioned instructions for preparing this Mediterranean dinner recipe:

1. Heat olive oil in a big heavy pot or Dutch Oven over medium heat until it only shimmers. Add the onions and raise the heat to medium-high temperatures. Saute for 5 minutes, frequently tossing.
2. Add garlic and all the vegetables that are chopped with salt and spices, season. To combine, toss.
3. Cook on medium-high heat for 5 to 7 minutes, frequently mixing with a wooden spoon.
4. Tomato, apricot and broth are added. With just a tiny dash of salt, season again.
5. Keep the heat on a medium-high and simmer for 10 minutes. Then reduce the heat for another 20 to 25 minutes or until the vegetables are soft, cover and simmer.

6. Stir in the chickpeas and cook on low heat for another 5 minutes.

7. Insert fresh parsley and lemon juice. Taste and change the seasoning to your liking, adding further salt or harissa spice blend.

8. Move to bowls for serving and finish each with a generous drizzle of extra virgin olive oil. Serve hot with your bread, couscous, or rice of choice. Enjoy.

24. Mediterranean Garlic Shrimp Pasta Recipe

Preparation time

20 minutes

Servings

4 persons

Nutritional facts

512.8 calories

Ingredients

We have listed below the ingredients that are required for making this dinner recipe:

- [Extra virgin olive oil](#)
- 1 lb large shrimp peeled and deveined (thawed if frozen)
- Black pepper
- Large handful chopped fresh parsley about One cup packed
- 2 to 3 vine ripe tomatoes chopped
- Parmesan cheese to your liking.
- ½ red onion chopped
- 5 garlic cloves minced
- 3/4 lb thin spaghetti
- Kosher salt
- One tsp dry oregano
- half teaspoon red pepper flakes (or One tsp [Aleppo pepper flakes](#))
- One cup dry white wine I used Pinot Grigio
- 1 lemon zested and juiced

Instructions

You need to follow the under mentioned instructions for preparing this Mediterranean dinner recipe:

1. Cook pasta according to the packet instructions in salted boiling water (about 9 minutes). Set aside a little bit of boiling water of the starchy pasta. Drain the pasta well.

2. Cook the shrimp as the pasta is cooking. One tbsp extra virgin olive oil is heated in a large pan at medium-high heat till the oil is shimmering but not smoking. For 2 to 3 minutes, cook the shrimp on either side until it turns yellow. For now, move the shrimp to a side dish.

3. In the same pan, if necessary, add a little more extra virgin olive oil. Decrease the heat to a medium-low level. Insert the onion, garlic, oregano and flakes of red pepper. Cook, stirring continuously, for 1 to 2 minutes. In the sauce, add the wine and scrape up any garlic and onion pieces. To reduce the volume, cook the wine for 1 minute, then insert the lemon juice and lemon zest.

4. Insert the chopped parsley and tomatoes and toss for 30 to 40 seconds or so. Season with Kosher salt.

5. Insert the cooked pasta into the pan and coat it with a toss. If you need to, insert some of the starchy pasta water.

6. Finally, add the shrimp that has been fried. Allow the shrimp to warm (another 30 seconds) for a short period, then remove the pasta from the heat.

7. Sprinkle with a little grated parmesan cheese as well as more red pepper flakes or Aleppo pepper to finish. Immediately serve.

25. Lemon Garlic Baked Chicken Drumsticks

Preparation time

1 hour 20 minutes

Servings

4 persons

Nutritional facts

143 calories

Ingredients

We have listed below the ingredients that are required for making this dinner recipe:

- 1 tablespoon dried oregano
- 1 tablespoon black pepper
- Zest &juice of two lemons + one lemon sliced
- Quarter cup extra virgin olive oil (Private Reserves Greek)
- 1 1/2 teaspoon coriander

- 1 teaspoon sweet paprika
- 1/2 teaspoon cumin
- 10 to 12 chicken drumsticks bone-in, skin on
- Kosher salt
- one garlic about twelve cloves of garlic, peeled & chopped
- one medium-sized yellow onion sliced into wedge.

Instructions

You need to follow the under mentioned instructions for preparing this Mediterranean dinner recipe:

1. Ensure to season underneath the skin as well after patting the chicken dry and seasoning with kosher salt. Arrange chicken on a tray or shallow dish if you have the time, & chill in the fridge for some hours or even overnight.

2. Place chicken in a big bag with a zip. Combine the spices (black pepper, paprika, oregano, coriander, and cumin) in a little bowl. Add spices in a bag with the chicken.

3. Insert the onion, garlic, lemon zest, olive oil and lemon juice. Zip up the bag. Toss the chicken around & rub it in the marinade to ensure it's well coated. Let chicken marinate for almost 30 mins, or refrigerate for two to four hours if you have the time.

4. Heat oven at 450 degrees f when ready.

5. Oil baking dish gently and arrange chicken drumsticks. In between, arrange the lemon slices.

6. Bake for about 35 mins or until chicken is cooked fully and the juices are clear. The chicken's internal temperature must register 165 degrees f . Broil for only a few mins if you like until the skin is crunchy to your taste.

26. Greek-Style Baked Cod Recipe with Lemon and Garlic

Preparation time

22 minutes

Servings

4 persons

Nutritional facts

312 calories

Ingredients

We have listed below the ingredients that are required for making this dinner recipe:

- Quarter cup chopped fresh parsley leaves

- 5 tbsp fresh lemon juice
- 3/4 tsp salt
- 1/2 tsp black pepper
- 5 tbsp Private Reserve extra virgin olive oil
- 1/3 cup all-purpose flour
- 1 tsp ground coriander
- 3/4 tsp sweet Spanish paprika
- 1.5 lb Cod fillet pieces (4-6 pieces)
- 5 garlic cloves, peeled and minced
- 3/4 tsp ground cumin

Instructions

You need to follow the under mentioned instructions for preparing this Mediterranean dinner recipe:

1. Heat oven to 400 degrees F.
2. In a shallow bowl, add the lemon juice, olive oil, and melted butter. Put aside.
3. Mix the all-purpose flour, spices, salt and pepper in another shallow bowl. Set next to the mixture of lemon juice.
4. Dry Pat Fish Fillet. Dip the fish in the mixture of lemon juice and then dip it in the mixture of flour. Shake the extra flour off. Reserve the mixture of lemon juice for later.
5. Heat a cast-iron skillet with two tablespoons of olive oil on medium-high heat. Ensure that oil shimmers and not smokes. To give it some flavor, add fish and sear on each side, but do not fully cook (about a couple of minutes on each side). Remove from heat.
6. The minced garlic and mix are added to the remaining lemon juice mixture. Drizzle over the fish fillets.
7. Bake in the hot oven until it starts to flake easily (10 minutes should do it, but begin checking earlier). Remove the chopped parsley from the heat and sprinkle.
8. Serving suggestions: Serve immediately with Lebanese rice and the typical Greek salad or this Mediterranean chickpea salad.

Conclusion

The Mediterranean diet focuses on the traditional foods that were consumed in 1960 in countries such as Italy and Greece. In comparison to Americans, these people were extremely healthy and had a comparatively low risk of several lifestyle diseases, according to the researchers. The Mediterranean diet has been related to a host of health benefits, including a healthier heart. A growing body of evidence suggests that the Mediterranean diet can help people lose weight and inhibit heart attacks, strokes, Type 2 diabetes, and premature death. The conventional healthy lifestyle habits of the people from the countries bordering the Mediterranean Sea, such as Greece, Italy, France, and Spain, are incorporated into a Mediterranean diet. Mediterranean diet has a variety of definitions because it varies by region and country. Fruits, vegetables, beans, legumes, nuts, grains, cereals, fish as well as unsaturated fats like olive oil are all abundant. It usually entails a restricted intake of dairy products and meat. You can incorporate more foods of Mediterranean-style into your diet by:

- Eating a variety of starchy foods, like bread and pasta, and • eating a variety of fruits and vegetables.
- Selecting products that have been made from plant and vegetable oils, like olive oil, in your diet
- Eating less meat

The Mediterranean diet closely resembles the government's healthier eating recommendations. A traditional Mediterranean diet includes plenty of fresh fruits and vegetables, whole grains, and legumes, as well as some healthy fats and fish. Below is a simple guide to help you select foods that are essential for a healthy, balanced diet, as well as how much of every food group you should consume:

- Base the meals on starchy foods like bread, potatoes, rice, & pasta – choose the wholegrain versions
- Eat the pulses or beans, eggs, meat, fish, & other proteins (like two portions of the fish per week, one of which must be oily)
- Have dairy or the dairy alteration

You don't have to achieve the balance with each meal, but over the course of a week or day, try to get it right. Unlike many other diets, the Mediterranean diet places a greater emphasis on plant foods. Whole grains, vegetables and legumes are frequently used to make up all or part of a meal. Cooking these foods with healthy fats like olive oil as well as plenty of flavorful spices is typical of people who follow the diet. Small portions of meat, fish, or eggs may be included in meals. Water, as well as sparkling water, are popular beverages.

www.ingramcontent.com/pod-product-compliance
Lightning Source LLC
Chambersburg PA
CBHW080629030426
42336CB00018B/3125